Study Guide and Procedure Checklist Manual for

Kinn's The Administrative Medical Assistant

An Applied Learning Approach

Fourteenth Edition

Brigitte Niedzwiecki, MSN, RN, RMA
Medical Assistant Program Director & Instructor
Chippewa Valley Technical College
Eau Claire, Wisconsin

Julie Pepper, BS, CMA (AAMA)
Medical Assistant Instructor
Chippewa Valley Technical College
Eau Claire, Wisconsin

P. Ann Weaver, MSEd, MT (ASCP)
Medical Assisting Instructor
Chippewa Valley Technical College
Eau Claire, Wisconsin

ELSEVIER

ELSEVIER

3251 Riverport Lane
St. Louis, Missouri 63043

Study Guide and Procedure Checklist Manual for
Kinn's The Administrative Medical Assistant, Fourteenth Edition   ISBN: 978-0-323-60836-7

ISBN: 978-0-323-60836-7

Printed in the United States of America

Last digit is the print number: 9 8 7 6 5 4 3 2 1

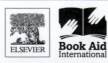

Working together
to grow libraries in
developing countries

www.elsevier.com • www.bookaid.org

To the Student

This study guide was created to help you to achieve the objectives of each chapter in your text and establish a solid base of knowledge in medical assisting. Completing the exercises in each chapter in this guide will help reinforce the material studied in the textbook and learned in class.

STUDY HINTS FOR ALL STUDENTS

Ask Questions!

There are no stupid questions. If you do not know something or are not sure about it, you need to find out. Other people may be wondering the same thing but are too shy to ask. The answer could be a matter of life or death for your patient. That is certainly more important than feeling embarrassed about asking a question.

Chapter Objectives

At the beginning of each chapter in the textbook are learning objectives that you should have mastered by the time you have finished studying that chapter. Write these objectives in your notebook, leaving a blank space after each. Fill in the answers as you find them while reading the chapter. Review to make sure your answers are correct and complete. Use these answers when you study for tests. You should also do this for separate course objectives that your instructor has listed in your class syllabus.

Vocabulary

At the beginning of each chapter in the textbook are vocabulary terms that you will encounter as you read the chapter. These terms are in bold type the first time they appear in the chapter.

Summary of Learning Objectives

Use the Summary of Learning Objectives at the end of each chapter in the textbook to help you review for exams.

Reading Hints

As you read each chapter in the textbook, look at the subject headings to learn what each section is about. Read first for the general meaning and then reread parts you did not understand. It may help to read those parts aloud. Carefully read the information given in each table and study each figure and its legend.

Concepts

While studying, put difficult concepts into your own words to determine whether you understand them. Check this understanding with another student or the instructor. Write these concepts in your notebook.

Class Notes

When taking lecture notes in class, leave a large margin on the left side of each notebook page and write only on right-hand pages, leaving all left-hand pages blank. Look over your lecture notes soon after each class while your memory is fresh. Fill in missing words, complete sentences and ideas, and underline key phrases, definitions, and concepts. At the top of each page, write the topic of that page. In the left margin, write the key word for that part of your notes. On the opposite left-hand page, write a summary or outline that combines material from the textbook and the lecture. These can be your study notes for review.

Study Groups

Form a study group with other students so that you can help one another. Practice speaking and reading aloud. Ask questions about material you find unclear. Work together to find answers.

ADDITIONAL STUDY HINTS FOR ENGLISH AS A SECOND LANGUAGE (ESL) STUDENTS

Vocabulary

If you find a nontechnical word you do not know (e.g., drowsy), try to guess its meaning from the sentence (e.g., with electrolyte imbalance, the patient may feel fatigued and drowsy). If you are not sure of the meaning or if it seems particularly important, look it up in the dictionary.

Vocabulary Notebook

Keep a small alphabetized notebook or address book in your pocket or purse. Write down new nontechnical words you read or hear along with their meanings and pronunciations. Write each word under its initial letter so you can find it easily, as with a dictionary. For words you do not know or words that have a different meaning in medical assisting, write down how each word is used and how it is pronounced. Look up the meanings of these words in a dictionary or ask your instructor or first-language buddy (see the following section). Then write the different meanings or uses that you have found in your book, including the medical assisting meaning. Continue to add new words as you discover them.

First-Language Buddy

English as a second language (ESL) students should find a first-language buddy—another student who is a native speaker of English and who is willing to answer questions about word meanings, pronunciations, and culture. Maybe, in turn, your buddy would like to learn about your language and culture; this could be useful for his or her medical assisting career.

Contents

Competency Checklist

Student Name: _____

Admission Cohort: _____

Graduation Date: _____

Competency	Procedure	Date	Grade / Pass	Initial
I. Anatomy & Physiology				
I.P.1.a. Measure and record: blood pressure				
I.P.1.b. Measure and record: temperature				
I.P.1.c. Measure and record: pulse				
I.P.1.d. Measure and record: respirations				
I.P.1.e. Measure and record: height				
I.P.1.f. Measure and record: weight				
I.P.1.g. Measure and record: length (infant)				
I.P.1.h. Measure and record: head circumference (infant)				
I.P.1.i. Measure and record: pulse oximetry				
I.P.2.a. Perform: electrocardiography				
I.P.2.b. Perform: venipuncture				
I.P.2.c. Perform: capillary puncture				
I.P.2.d. Perform: pulmonary function testing				
I.P.3. Perform patient screening using established protocols				
I.P.4.a. Verify the rules of medication administration: right patient				
I.P.4.b. Verify the rules of medication administration: right medication				
I.P.4.c. Verify the rules of medication administration: right dose				
I.P.4.d. Verify the rules of medication administration: right route				
I.P.4.e. Verify the rules of medication administration: right time				

Competency	Procedure	Date	Grade / Pass	Initial
I.P.4.f. Verify the rules of medication administration: right documentation				
I.P.5. Select proper sites for administering parenteral medication				
I.P.6. Administer oral medications				
I.P.7. Administer parenteral (excluding IV) medications				
I.P.8. Instruct and prepare a patient for a procedure or a treatment				
I.P.9. Assist provider with a patient exam				
I.P.10. Perform a quality control measure				
I.P.11.a. Obtain specimens and perform: CLIA-waived hematology test				
I.P.11.b. Obtain specimens and perform: CLIA-waived chemistry test				
I.P.11.c. Obtain specimens and perform: CLIA-waived urinalysis				
I.P.11.d. Obtain specimens and perform: CLIA-waived immunology test				
I.P.11.e. Obtain specimens and perform: CLIA-waived microbiology test				
I.P.12. Produce up-to-date documentation of provider/ professional level CPR				
I.P.13.a. Perform first aid procedures for: bleeding	Procedure 21-5			
I.P.13.b. Perform first aid procedures for: diabetic coma or insulin shock	Procedure 21-1			
I.P.13.c. Perform first aid procedures for: fractures	Procedure 21-5			
I.P.13.d. Perform first aid procedures for: seizures	Procedure 21-3			
I.P.13.e. Perform first aid procedures for: shock	Procedure 21-6			
I.P.13.f. Perform first aid procedures for: syncope	Procedure 21-5			
I.A.1. Incorporate critical thinking skills when performing patient assessment	Procedure 21-2			

Competency	Procedure	Date	Grade / Pass	Initial
I.A.2. Incorporate critical thinking skills when performing patient care				
I.A.3. Show awareness of a patient's concerns related to the procedure being performed				
II. Applied Mathematics				
II.P.1. Calculate proper dosages of medication for administration				
II.P.2. Differentiate between normal and abnormal test results				
II.P.3. Maintain lab test results using flow sheets				
II.P.4. Document on a growth chart				
II.A.1. Reassure a patient of the accuracy of the test results				
III. Infection Control				
III.P.1. Participate in bloodborne pathogen training				
III.P.2. Select appropriate barrier/ personal protective equipment (PPE)				
III.P.3. Perform hand washing				
III.P.4. Prepare items for autoclaving				
III.P.5. Perform sterilization procedures				
III.P.6. Prepare a sterile field				
III.P.7. Perform within a sterile field				
III.P.8. Perform wound care				
III.P.9. Perform dressing change				
III.P.10.a. Demonstrate proper disposal of biohazardous material: sharps				
III.P.10.b. Demonstrate proper disposal of biohazardous material: regulated wastes				
III.A.1. Recognize the implications for failure to comply with Center for Disease Control (CDC) regulations in healthcare settings				
IV. Nutrition				
IV.P.1. Instruct a patient according to patient's special dietary needs				
IV.A.1. Show awareness of patient's concerns regarding a dietary change				

Competency	Procedure	Date	Grade / Pass	Initial
V. Concepts of Effective Communication				
V.P.1.a. Use feedback techniques to obtain patient information including: reflection	Procedures 2-1, 2-2, 2-4			
V.P.1.b. Use feedback techniques to obtain patient information including: restatement	Procedures 2-1, 2-2, 2-4			
V.P.1.c. Use feedback techniques to obtain patient information including: clarification	Procedures 2-1, 2-2, 2-4			
V.P.2. Respond to nonverbal communication	Procedures 2-1 to 2-4			
V.P.3. Use medical terminology correctly and pronounced accurately to communicate information to providers and patients				
V.P.4.a. Coach patients regarding: office policies	Procedure 11-3			
V.P.4.b. Coach patients regarding: health maintenance				
V.P.4.c. Coach patients regarding: disease prevention	Procedure 7-1			
V.P.4.d. Coach patients regarding: treatment plan				
V.P.5.a. Coach patients appropriately considering: cultural diversity				
V.P.5.b. Coach patients appropriately considering: developmental life stage	Procedure 7-1			
V.P.5.c. Coach patients appropriately considering: communication barriers	Procedure 7-1			
V.P.6. Demonstrate professional telephone techniques	Procedure 10-1			
V.P.7. Document telephone messages accurately	Procedure 10-2			
V.P.8. Compose professional correspondence utilizing electronic technology	Procedures 9-1 to 9-5			
V.P.9. Develop a current list of community resources related to patients' healthcare needs	Procedure 7-2			
V.P.10. Facilitate referrals to community resources in the role of a patient navigator	Procedure 7-2			

Competency	Procedure	Date	Grade / Pass	Initial
V.P.11. Report relevant information concisely and accurately	Procedure 10-2			
V.A.1.a. Demonstrate: empathy	Procedures 2-1 to 2-4			
V.A.1.b. Demonstrate: active listening	Procedures 2-1 to 2-4			
V.A.1.c. Demonstrate: nonverbal communication	Procedures 2-1 to 2-4			
V.A.2. Demonstrate the principles of self-boundaries				
V.A.3.a. Demonstrate respect for individual diversity including: gender	Procedure 2-1			
V.A.3.b. Demonstrate respect for individual diversity including: race	Procedure 2-2			
V.A.3.c. Demonstrate respect for individual diversity including: religion	Procedure 2-3			
V.A.3.d. Demonstrate respect for individual diversity including: age	Procedure 2-4			
V.A.3.e. Demonstrate respect for individual diversity including: economic status	Procedure 2-4			
V.A.3.f. Demonstrate respect for individual diversity including: appearance	Procedures 2-1 to 2-4			
V.A.4. Explain to a patient the rationale for performance of a procedure				
VI. Administrative Functions				
VI.P.1. Manage appointment schedule using established priorities	Procedures 11-1, 11-2, 11-4			
VI.P.2. Schedule a patient procedure	Procedure 11-5			
VI.P.3. Create a patient's medical record	Procedures 12-1, 12-4			
VI.P.4. Organize a patient's medical record	Procedures 12-2, 12-4			
VI.P.5. File patient medical records	Procedures 12-2, 12-4, 12-5			
VI.P.6. Utilize an EMR	Procedure 12-2			
VI.P.7. Input patient data utilizing a practice management system	Procedures 12-1, 12-2			
VI.P.8. Perform routine maintenance of administrative or clinical equipment	Procedure 13-2			
VI.P.9. Perform an inventory with documentation	Procedures 13-1, 13-3			
VI.A.1. Display sensitivity when managing appointments	Procedures 11-2, 11-4, 11-5			

Competency	Procedure	Date	Grade / Pass	Initial
VII. Basic Practice Finances				
VII.P.1.a. Perform accounts receivable procedures to patient accounts including posting: charges	Procedure 19-1			
VII.P.1.b. Perform accounts receivable procedures to patient accounts including posting: payments	Procedures 19-1, 19-3			
VII.P.1.c. Perform accounts receivable procedures to patient accounts including posting: adjustments	Procedure 19-3			
VII.P.2. Prepare a bank deposit	Procedure 19-4			
VII.P.3. Obtain accurate patient billing information	Procedure 11-2 Procedure 19-2			
VII.P.4. Inform a patient of financial obligations for services rendered	Procedure 18-6 Procedure 19-2			
VII.A.1. Demonstrate professionalism when discussing patient's billing record	Procedures 18-2, 18-6 Procedure 19-2			
VII.A.2. Display sensitivity when requesting payment for services rendered	Procedures 18-2, 18-6 Procedure 19-2			
VIII. Third Party Reimbursement				
VIII.P.1. Interpret information on an insurance card	Procedure 15-1 Procedure 18-1			
VIII.P.2. Verify eligibility for services including documentation	Procedure 15-2 Procedure 18-6			
VIII.P.3. Obtain precertification or preauthorization including documentation	Procedure 15-2 Procedure 18-3			
VIII.P.4. Complete an insurance claim form	Procedure 18-4			
VIII.A.1. Interact professionally with third party representatives	Procedure 18-2			
VIII.A.2. Display tactful behavior when communicating with medical providers regarding third party requirements	Procedure 18-2			
VIII.A.3. Show sensitivity when communicating with patients regarding third party requirements	Procedure 18-2			
IX. Procedural and Diagnostic Coding				
IX.P.1. Perform procedural coding	Procedures 17-1, 17-2			
IX.P.2. Perform diagnostic coding	Procedure 16-1			

Competency	Procedure	Date	Grade / Pass	Initial
IX.P.3. Utilize medical necessity guidelines	Procedure 18-5			
IX.A.1. Utilize tactful communication skills with medical providers to ensure accurate code selection	Procedure 17-3			
X. Legal Implications				
X.P.1. Locate a state's legal scope of practice for medical assistants	Procedure 3-2			
X.P.2.a. Apply HIPAA rules in regard to: privacy	Procedure 4-1			
X.P.2.b. Apply HIPAA rules in regard to: release of information	Procedure 4-2			
X.P.3. Document patient care accurately in the medical record	Procedures 7-1, 7-2 Procedures 21-1 to 21-6			
X.P.4.a. Apply the Patient's Bill of Rights as it relates to: choice of treatment	Procedure 3-1			
X.P.4.b. Apply the Patient's Bill of Rights as it relates to: consent for treatment	Procedure 3-1			
X.P.4.c. Apply the Patient's Bill of Rights as it relates to: refusal of treatment	Procedure 3-1			
X.P.5. Perform compliance reporting based on public health statutes	Procedure 4-3			
X.P.6. Report an illegal activity in the healthcare setting following proper protocol	Procedure 4-4			
X.P.7. Complete an incident report related to an error in patient care	Procedure 4-5			
X.A.1. Demonstrate sensitivity to patient rights	Procedure 3-1 Procedure 4-1			
X.A.2. Protect the integrity of the medical record	Procedures 12-1 to 12-3			
XI. Ethical Considerations				
XI.P.1. Develop a plan for separation of personal and professional ethics	Procedure 5-1			
XI.P.2. Demonstrate appropriate response(s) to ethical issues	Procedure 5-2			
XI.A.1. Recognize the impact personal ethics and morals have on the delivery of healthcare	Procedure 5-1, 5-2			

Competency	Procedure	Date	Grade / Pass	Initial
XII. Protective Practices				
XII.P.1.a. Comply with: safety signs				
XII.P.1.b. Comply with: symbols				
XII.P.1.c. Comply with: labels				
XII.P.2.a. Demonstrate proper use of: eyewash equipment				
XII.P.2.b. Demonstrate proper use of: fire extinguishers	Procedure 13-6			
XII.P.2.c. Demonstrate proper use of: sharps disposal containers				
XII.P.3. Use proper body mechanics	Procedure 13-4			
XII.P.4. Participate in a mock exposure event with documentation of specific steps	Procedure 13-5			
XII.P.5. Evaluate the work environment to identify unsafe working conditions	Procedure 13-4			
XII.A.1. Recognize the physical and emotional effects on persons involved in an emergency situation	Procedure 13-5			
XII.A.2. Demonstrate self-awareness in responding to an emergency situation	Procedure 13-5			

The Professional Medical Assistant and the Healthcare Team

CAAHEP Competencies	Assessments
V.C.12. Define patient navigator	Workplace Application – 2
V.C.13. Describe the role of the medical assistant as a patient navigator	Workplace Application – 2
VIII.C.4. Define a patient-centered medical home (PCMH)	Skills and Concepts – J. 1
X.C.1. Differentiate between scope of practice and standards of care for medical assistants	Skills and Concepts – C. 1
X.C.2. Compare and contrast provider and medical assistant roles in terms of standard of care	Skills and Concepts – C. 2
V.C.11. Define the principles of self-boundaries	Skills and Concepts – K. 2
ABHES Competencies	**Assessments**
1. General Orientation a. Describe the current employment outlook for the medical assistant	Skills and Concepts – A. 1, 2
b. Compare and contrast the allied health professions and understand their relation to medical assisting	Skills and Concepts – H. 1-19
c. Describe and comprehend medical assistant credentialing requirements, the process to obtain the credential and the importance of credentialing	Skills and Concepts – D. 1
d. List the general responsibilities and skills of the medical assistant	Skills and Concepts – A. 3
5. Human Relations f. Demonstrate an understanding of the core competencies for Interprofessional Collaborative Practice i.e. values/ethics; roles/responsibilities; interprofessional communication; teamwork	Skills and Concepts – J. 2
g. Partner with health care teams to attain optimal patient health outcomes	Skills and Concepts – K. 1
h. Display effective interpersonal skills with patients and health care team members	Skills and Concepts – K. 1
i. Demonstrate cultural awareness	Skills and Concepts – B. 1

ABHES Competencies	Assessments
8. Clinical Procedures i. Identify community resources and Complementary and Alternative Medicine practices (CAM)	Skills and Concepts – G. 3

VOCABULARY REVIEW

Using the word pool on the right, find the correct word to match the definition. Write the word on the line after the definition.

Group A

1. Adhering to ethical standards or right conduct standards _____

2. The way an individual perceives and processes information to learn new material _____

3. To learn or memorize beyond the point of proficiency or immediate recall _____

4. The process of sorting patients to determine medical need and the priority of care _____

5. A person who identifies patients' needs and barriers, then assists by coordinating care and identifying community and healthcare resources to meet the needs _____

6. How an individual internalizes new information and makes it his or her own _____

7. A learning device (e.g., an image, a rhyme, or a figure of speech) that a person uses to help him or her remember information _____

8. Meticulous, careful _____

9. How an individual looks at information and sees it as real _____

10. The process of thinking about new information to create new ways of learning _____

11. Harmful _____

12. Conduct expected of a reasonably prudent person acting under similar circumstances; it falls below the standards of behavior established by law for the protection of others against unreasonable risk of harm _____

Word Pool
- patient navigator
- detrimental
- integrity
- conscientious
- triage
- negligence
- perceiving
- processing
- learning style
- reflection
- overlearn
- mnemonic

Group B

1. A group of diverse medical and healthcare systems, practices, and products that are not generally considered part of conventional medicine. Some are used in combination with conventional medicine and others are used instead of conventional medicine

   _____

2. Emotional or mental condition with respect to cheerfulness or confidence _____

3. A system of medical practice that treats disease by the use of remedies such as medications and surgery to produce effects different from those caused by the disease under treatment

   _____

4. Dependable, able to be trusted _____

5. The process by which something becomes harmful or unusable through contact with something unclean

   _____

6. The ability to determine what needs to be done and take action on your own _____

7. A form of healing that considers the whole person (i.e., body, mind, spirit, and emotions) in individual treatment plans

   _____

8. A concept of care that involves health professionals and volunteers who provide medical, psychological, and spiritual support to terminally ill patients and their loved ones

   _____

9. Behavior toward others; outward manner

   _____

10. The constant practice of considering all aspects of a situation when deciding what to believe or what to do

    _____

11. An important point or group of statistical values that, when evaluated, indicates the quality of care provided in a healthcare facility _____

Word Pool
- critical thinking
- contamination
- allopathic
- holistic
- complementary and alternative medicine (CAM)
- hospice
- indicators
- demeanor
- initiative
- reliable
- morale

ABBREVIATIONS

Write out what each of the following abbreviations stands for.

1. CAAHEP _____

2. CAM _____

3. EHR _____

4. ECG _____

5. CLIA _____

6. OSHA _____

7. IV _____

8. AAMA _____

9. CEU _____

10. AMT _____

11. NHA _____

12. MD _____

13. DO _____

14. OMT _____

15. DC _____

16. NP _____

17. RN _____

18. PA _____

19. IDS _____

20. ED _____

21. PCMH _____

22. AHRQ _____

23. HHS _____

24. IT _____

SKILLS AND CONCEPTS

Answer the following questions. Write your answer on the line or in the space provided.

A. Responsibilities of the Medical Assistant

1. According the U.S. Bureau of Labor Statistics, employment opportunities for medical assistants is expected to grow _____ through _____ .

2. List factors for the expected growth in job opportunities for medical assistants. _____

_____

_____

_____

_____

_____

_____

3. List five clinical and five administrative skills that are part of the job description for an entry-level medical assistant.

   Clinical skills include: _____

   _____

   _____

   _____

   _____

   _____

   Administrative skills include: _____

   _____

   _____

   _____

   _____

   _____

B. Characteristics of Professional Medical Assistants

1. What methods can the medical assistant use to treat others with courtesy and respect? _____

   _____

   _____

   _____

   _____

   _____

C. Scope of Practice and Standards of Care for Medical Assistants

1. What is the difference between scope of practice and standards of care? _____

   _____

   _____

   _____

   _____

   _____

2. Describe the difference between standard of care for a provider and a medical assistant._____

_____

_____

_____

_____

_____

3. Identify five practices that are beyond the scope of practice of medical assistants._____

_____

_____

_____

_____

_____

D. Professional Medical Assisting Organizations, Credentials, and Continuing Education

1. What are some of the differences between the AAMA and AMT? What credentials can be granted by each?

_____

_____

_____

_____

_____

_____

2. Is the NHA involved in medical assistant program curriculum development or accreditation? What service does this company provide?

_____

_____

_____

_____

_____

_____

E. How to Succeed as a Medical Assistant Student

1. Choose three study skills from your reading and describe how you think they will help you learn.

    _____

    _____

    _____

    _____

    _____

2. What test-taking strategies might help you improve your scores?_____

    _____

    _____

    _____

3. Describe what it means to be a critical thinker. _____

    _____

    _____

    _____

    _____

    _____

F. The History of Medicine

1. Describe how the profession of medical assisting began. Why are medical assistants defined as *multi-skilled* healthcare workers?

    _____

    _____

    _____

    _____

    _____

G. Medical Professionals

1. _____ physicians, or DOs, complete requirements similar to those for MDs to graduate and practice medicine.

2. _____ provide direct patient care services under the supervision of licensed physicians and are trained to diagnose and treat patients as directed by the physician.

I. Types of Healthcare Facilities

1. Hospitals are classified according to the type of care and services they provide to patients. Describe the three different levels of hospitalized care.

    a. _____

    _____

    _____

    _____

    b. _____

    _____

    _____

    _____

    c. _____

    _____

    _____

    _____

J. The Healthcare Team

1. Define a patient-centered medical home (PCMH) and its five core functions and attributes. _____

    _____

    _____

    _____

    _____

    _____

    _____

    _____

2. Define teamwork in your own words._____

    _____

    _____

    _____

    _____

    _____

K. Professionalism as a Team Member

1. Summarize three obstructions to professionalism.

    a. _____

    _____

    _____

    _____

    b. _____

    _____

    _____

    _____

    c. _____

    _____

    _____

    _____

2. Define the principles of self-boundaries. How do they relate to the field of medical assisting? _____

    _____

    _____

    _____

    _____

    _____

    _____

    _____

3. Describe four time-management techniques medical assistants can use in the healthcare environment to meet the demands of a busy practice.

    a. _____

    b. _____

    c. _____

    d. _____

CERTIFICATION PREPARATION

Circle the correct answer.

1. The first national organization formed for medical assistants was the
   a. CAAHEP.
   b. ABHES.
   c. AMT.
   d. AAMA.

2. Which healthcare professional is trained to practice medicine under the supervision of a physician?
   a. Medical technologist
   b. Paramedic
   c. Medical assistant
   d. Physician assistant

3. The allied health specialist who performs ultrasound diagnostic procedures under the supervision of a physician is called a(n)
   a. cytotechnologist.
   b. diagnostic medical sonographer.
   c. electroneurodiagnostic technologist.
   d. perfusionist.

4. A method of prioritizing patients so that the most urgent cases receive care first is called
   a. case management.
   b. accreditation.
   c. triage.
   d. quality control.

5. The health professional who provides basic patient care services, including diagnosing illnesses and prescribing medications, is a
   a. nurse practitioner.
   b. nurse anesthetist.
   c. licensed practical nurse.
   d. vocational nurse.

6. One factor is absolutely true about all practicing medical assistants—they are not independent practitioners. Whether certified or not, regardless of length of training or experience, every medical assistant must practice under the direct supervision of a physician or other licensed practitioner (e.g., nurse practitioner or physician assistant).
   a. Both statements are true.
   b. Both statements are false.
   c. The first statement is true; the second is false.
   d. The first statement is false; the second is true.

7. Which mind maps would display the cause and effect of events?
   a. Spider map
   b. Fishbone map
   c. Chain-of-events map
   d. Cycle map

8. Which is *not* part of critical thinking?
   a. Sorting out conflicting information
   b. Weighing your knowledge about the information
   c. Deciding on a reasonable belief or action
   d. Incorporating personal beliefs

9. Deciding which tasks are most important is called
   a. modification.
   b. teaching.
   c. prioritizing.
   d. procrastinating.

10. Which statement about professionalism is true?
    a. It must be practiced at all times in the workplace.
    b. It can lead to wage increases and promotions.
    c. Unacceptable behavior is detrimental to the medical assistant's career.
    d. All of the above are true.

WORKPLACE APPLICATIONS

1. You are employed by a primary care physician who is investigating the possibility of forming a PCMH with other practitioners and allied health professionals in the community. Refer to the Department of Health and Human Services PCMH Resource Center at http://pcmh.ahrq.gov/. Research the meaning of PCMH and review the research that supports the PCMH model of care. What did you learn? Share this information with your class.

2. What does it mean to operate as a patient navigator? Why are medical assistants who are skilled in both administrative and clinical areas ideally suited to help patients navigate complex healthcare systems? How could you help the patient described below?

   Mrs. Kate Glasgow is an 82-year-old patient in the family practice where you work. Mrs. Glasgow recently suffered a mild cerebrovascular accident (CVA) and her son is trying to help coordinate her care. Mrs. Glasgow does not understand when or how to take her new medications, she is concerned about whether her health insurance will cover the cost of frequent clinic appointments and assistive devices, she doesn't understand how to prepare for magnetic resonance imaging (MRI) the provider ordered, and she dislikes having to comply with getting blood drawn every week.

3. Martin Smith is a patient who always disrupts the clinic. He constantly complains about everything from the moment he enters until the moment he leaves. Karen is at the desk when he arrives to check out and pay his bill. When she tells him that he has a previous balance from a claim that his insurance did not pay, he argues that Karen filed the claim incorrectly. Karen is not in charge of filing insurance claims and did not handle any part of the claim in question. How can she be courteous to this patient?

INTERNET ACTIVITIES

1. Choose one of the early medical pioneers discussed in this chapter and research him or her using the internet. After conducting the research, create a poster presentation, a PowerPoint presentation, or write a paper and present the results of your research to the class.

2. Research professionalism requirements for other health professions. Talk about the ways that those requirements are similar to or different from those of a medical assistant. Compare professionalism in the healthcare industry to that in other professions, such as law enforcement or education. Talk about why medical professionalism is so critical.

Therapeutic Communication

CAAHEP Competencies	Assessment
V.C.1. Identify styles and types of verbal communication	Skills and Concepts – D. 1, 4-9; Certification Preparation – 2
V.C.2. Identify types of nonverbal communication	Skills and Concepts – C. 2-5; Certification Preparation – 1
V.C.3. Recognize barriers to communication	Skills and Concepts – D. 21 a-h; Certification Preparation – 3
V.C.4. Identify techniques for overcoming communication barriers	Skills and Concepts – D. 22 a-h; Certification Preparation – 4
V.C.5. Recognize the elements of oral communication using a sender-receiver process	Skills and Concepts – D. 2-3
V.C.14.a. Relate the following behaviors to professional communication: assertive	Skills and Concepts – D. 9 a-e, 10
V.C.14.b. Relate the following behaviors to professional communication: aggressive	Skills and Concepts – D. 6 a-e
V.C.14.c. Relate the following behaviors to professional communication: passive	Skills and Concepts – D. 5 a-e
V.C.15. Differentiate between adaptive and non-adaptive coping mechanisms	Skills and Concepts – E. 6-8; Certification Preparation – 5; Internet Activities – 4
V.C.18.a. Discuss examples of diversity: cultural	Skills and Concepts – B. 1
V.C.18.b. Discuss examples of diversity: social	Skills and Concepts – B. 2
V.C.18.c. Discuss examples of diversity: ethnic	Skills and Concepts – B. 3
V.A.3.a. Demonstrate respect for individual diversity including: gender	Procedure 2.1
V.A.3.b. Demonstrate respect for individual diversity including: race	Procedure 2.2
V.A.3.c. Demonstrate respect for individual diversity including: religion	Procedure 2.3
V.A.3.d. Demonstrate respect for individual diversity including: age	Procedure 2.4
V.A.3.e. Demonstrate respect for individual diversity including: economic status	Procedure 2.4

CAAHEP Competencies	Assessment
V.A.3.f. Demonstrate respect for individual diversity including: appearance	Procedure 2.1, 2.2, 2.3, 2.4
V.P.1.a. Use feedback techniques to obtain patient information including: reflection	Procedure 2.1, 2.2, 2.4
V.P.1.b. Use feedback techniques to obtain patient information including: restatement	Procedure 2.1, 2.2, 2.4
V.P.1.c. Use feedback techniques to obtain patient information including: clarification	Procedure 2.1, 2.2, 2.4
V.P.2. Respond to nonverbal communication	Procedure 2.1, 2.2, 2.3, 2.4
V.A.1.a. Demonstrate: empathy	Procedure 2.1, 2.2, 2.3, 2.4
V.A.1.b. Demonstrate: active listening	Procedure 2.1, 2.2, 2.3, 2.4
V.A.1.c. Demonstrate: nonverbal communication	Procedure 2.1, 2.2, 2.3, 2.4
V.C.17.a. Discuss the theories of: Maslow	Skills and Concepts – E. 1, 2 a-e; Certification Preparation – 8-9; Internet Activities – 3
V.C.17.b. Discuss the theories of: Erikson	Skills and Concepts – D. 23, 24 a-i; Certification Preparation – 6
V.C.17.c. Discuss the theories of: Kübler-Ross	Skills and Concepts – D. 25, 26 a-e; Certification Preparation – 7
V.C.11. Define the principles of self-boundaries	Skills and Concepts – D. 27
X.C.10.c. Identify: Americans with Disabilities Act Amendments Act (ADAAA)	Skills and Concepts – F. 1

ABHES Competencies	Assessment
5. Human Relations a. Respond appropriately to patients with abnormal behavior patterns	Skills and Concepts – E. 4
b. Provide support for terminally ill patients 1) Use empathy when communicating with terminally ill patients	Procedure 2.4
b. 2) Identify common stages that terminally ill patients experience	Skills and Concepts – D. 25, 26 a-e
e. Analyze the effect of hereditary and environmental influences on behavior	Skills and Concepts – E. 1-3
i . Display effective interpersonal skills with patients and health care team members	Procedure 2.1, 2.2, 2.3, 2.4

VOCABULARY REVIEW

Using the word pool on the right, find the correct word to match the definition. Write the word on the line after the definition.

1. The ability to understand another's perspective, experiences, or motivations _____

2. The act of sticking to something _____

3. A type of communication that occurs through body language and expressive behaviors rather than with verbal or written words

   _____

4. The inherent worth or state of being worthy of respect

   _____

5. Having a deep awareness of the suffering of another and the wish to ease it _____

6. The differences and similarities in identity, perspective, and points of view among people _____

7. Having a composed and self-assured manner

   _____

8. A relationship of harmony and accord between the patient and the healthcare professional _____

9. To show consideration or appreciation for another person

   _____

10. A condition that causes physical and/or emotional tension

    _____

11. Exchange of information, feelings, and thoughts between two or more people using spoken words or other methods

    _____

12. A process of communicating with patients and family members in healthcare _____

13. Things arranged in order or rank _____

14. Unconscious mental processes that protect people from anxiety, loss, conflict, or shame _____

15. Behavioral and psychological strategies used to deal with or minimize stressful events _____

Word Pool
- respect
- dignity
- empathy
- compassion
- adherence
- stress
- nonverbal communication
- communication
- therapeutic communication
- coping mechanisms
- hierarchy
- defense mechanisms
- rapport
- poised
- diversity

ABBREVIATIONS

Write out what each of the following abbreviations stands for.

1. ADA _____

2. ADAAA _____

SKILLS AND CONCEPTS

Answer the following questions. Write your answer on the line or in the space provided.

A. First Impressions

1. _____ is a process of communicating with patients and family members in healthcare.

2. What factors are involved in creating a first impression? _____

   _____

   _____

   _____

B. Diversity and Communication

1. Describe cultural diversity and discuss two examples. _____

   _____

   _____

2. Describe social diversity and discuss two examples. _____

   _____

   _____

3. Describe ethnic diversity and discuss two examples. _____

   _____

   _____

4. Describe when a medical assistant must respect individual diversity and why is this important.

   _____

   _____

   _____

5. How does a medical assistant respect another's diversity? What should the medical assistant do or not do?

   _____

   _____

6. Describe why it is important to address diversity biases prior to providing patient care. _____

   _____

   _____

C. Nonverbal Communication

1. What is the importance of nonverbal communication? _____

    _____

    _____

2. Describe the three types of nonverbal communication. _____

    _____

    _____

3. List five types of nonverbal behavior. _____

    _____

    _____

4. Describe positive and open nonverbal behaviors that should be used with patients._____

    _____

    _____

    _____

5. List 10 nonverbal communication delivery factors._____

    _____

    _____

    _____

    _____

6. If you are working with a patient from another cultural group that you are unfamiliar with, describe three tips to follow.

    _____

    _____

    _____

7. When medical assistants talk with patients, they should be _____ away from the patients, which is considered the _____ space.

8. When medical assistants perform procedures on patients, they are _____ away from patients, which is considered the _____ space.

9. What is one action people take when they want to increase the space between themselves and other people?

    _____

    _____

10. What are three actions people take when they want to decrease the space between themselves and other people?

_____

_____

_____

D. Verbal Communication

1. What are the two types of verbal communication? _____

_____

2. Describe the parts of the communication cycle. _____

_____

_____

3. We decode messages based on _____ and _____.

4. List three types of written communication. _____

_____

5. Describe passive communicators.

   a. Description of communication: _____

   _____

   _____

   b. Nonverbal communication behaviors used: _____

   _____

   _____

   c. How they may feel: _____

   _____

   _____

   d. How others may feel with this behavior: _____

   _____

   _____

   e. Based on what you learned about this type of communicator, how would you professionally communicate with this type of person?

   _____

   _____

6. Describe aggressive communicators.

   a. Description of communication: _____

      _____

      _____

   b. Nonverbal communication behaviors used: _____

      _____

      _____

   c. How they may feel: _____

      _____

      _____

   d. How others may feel with this behavior:_____

      _____

      _____

   e. Based on what you learned about this type of communicator, how would you professionally communicate with this type of person?

      _____

      _____

7. Describe passive-aggressive communicators.

   a. Description of communication: _____

      _____

      _____

   b. Nonverbal communication behaviors used: _____

      _____

      _____

   c. How they may feel: _____

      _____

      _____

   d. How others may feel with this behavior:_____

      _____

      _____

e.   Based on what you learned about this type of communicator, how would you professionally communicate with this type of person?

_____

_____

8.   Describe manipulative communicators.

a.   Description of communication: _____

_____

_____

b.   Nonverbal communication behaviors used: _____

_____

_____

c.   How they may feel: _____

_____

_____

d.   How others may feel with this behavior: _____

_____

_____

e.   Based on what you learned about this type of communicator, how would you professionally communicate with this type of person?

_____

_____

9.   Describe assertive communicators.

a.   Description of communication: _____

_____

_____

b.   Nonverbal communication behaviors used: _____

_____

_____

c.   How they may feel: _____

_____

_____

    d. How others may feel with this behavior: _____

_____

_____

    e. Based on what you learned about this type of communicator, how would you professionally communicate with this type of person?

_____

_____

10. What type of communicator should a medical assistant strive to become? Explain why this type of communicator is important in a healthcare setting.

_____

_____

_____

11. What are the advantages of using therapeutic communication in a healthcare setting? _____

_____

_____

_____

12. Describe the difference between active listening and passively hearing what the speaker is saying.

_____

_____

_____

13. List four nonverbal behaviors that can be used during active listening. _____

_____

_____

14. Describe open questions or statements and identify when to use them with patients. _____

_____

_____

_____

15. Describe closed questions or statements and identify when to use them with patients. _____

_____

_____

_____

16. _____ allows the listener to get additional information.

17. _____ or _____ means to reword or rephrase a statement to check the meaning and interpretation.

18. _____ allows the listener to recap and review what was said.

19. _____ allows time to gather thoughts and answer questions.

20. _____ means to put words to the person's emotional reaction, which acknowledges the person's feelings.

21. For each description below, identify the type of barrier to communication.

   a. Noise, lack of privacy, temperature: _____

   b. Fear and anxiety related to being judged by the healthcare professional or the inability to explain personal feelings: _____

   c. Unable to read or write: _____

   d. Hunger, pain, anger, tiredness: _____

   e. Unable to see written communication: _____

   f. Unable to hear verbal communication: _____

   g. Functioning at a lower age level: _____

   h. English is not the patient's primary language: _____

22. Describe ways the medical assistant can help overcome barriers to communication.

   a. Internal distractions: _____

   _____

   _____

   b. Visual impairment: _____

   _____

   _____

   c. Hearing impairment: _____

   _____

   _____

   d. Environmental distractions: _____

   _____

   _____

   e. Illiteracy: _____

   _____

   _____

    f.   Non-English–speaking:_____

              _____

              _____

    g.   Intellectual disability: _____

              _____

              _____

    h.   Emotional distraction:_____

              _____

              _____

23. Discuss how Erikson's theory of psychosocial developmental relates to communicating with patients.

      _____

      _____

      _____

24. Discuss Erikson's psychosocial developmental stages. Your answers should include the goals of the stage and one communication tip for that stage.

    a.   Trust versus Mistrust: _____

              _____

              _____

              _____

    b.   Autonomy versus Shame and Doubt: _____

              _____

              _____

              _____

    c.   Initiative versus Guilt:_____

              _____

              _____

              _____

    d.   Industry versus Inferiority: _____

              _____

              _____

              _____

e.   Identity versus Role Confusion: _____

_____

_____

_____

f.   Intimacy versus Isolation:_____

_____

_____

_____

g.   Generativity versus Stagnation: _____

_____

_____

_____

h.   Ego Integrity versus Despair: _____

_____

_____

_____

25. Discuss how Kübler-Ross's theory relates to communicating with patients. _____

_____

_____

_____

26. Describe the following stages of Kübler-Ross's theory.

a.   Denial: _____

_____

_____

b.   Anger: _____

_____

_____

c.   Bargaining: _____

_____

_____

    d. Depression: _____

_____

_____

    e. Acceptance: _____

_____

_____

27. Based on the principles of personal boundaries, describe three ways communication with patients differs from communication with family and friends.

_____

_____

_____

_____

_____

_____

_____

_____

E. Understanding Behavior

1.   Describe Maslow's Hierarchy of Needs theory. _____

_____

_____

_____

_____

_____

2.   For the following descriptions, identify the level of need according to Maslow's theory.

    a. Includes air, food, drink, shelter, and warmth: _____

    b. Includes friendship and intimacy: _____

    c. Includes protection form the elements and security: _____

    d. Includes knowledge, curiosity, and understanding: _____

    e. The appreciation of and search for beauty and balance: _____

    f. Includes self-esteem and achievement: _____

    g. The need to realize one's potential: _____

    h. These needs are met by helping others achieve their very best: _____

3. Describe how understanding Maslow's theory can help a medical assistant. _____

_____

_____

4. Why do people use defense mechanisms? _____

_____

_____

5. Identify the defense mechanism based on the following descriptions.

   a. Completely rejects the information: _____

   b. The person comes up with various explanations to justify his or her response:

      _____

   c. Transfers the emotion toward one person to another person or thing: _____

   d. Simply forgets something that is bad or hurtful: _____

6. Describe the difference between adaptive (healthy) coping mechanisms and maladaptive (nonadaptive or unhealthy) coping mechanisms.

   _____

   _____

   _____

7. List four adaptive coping mechanisms._____

   _____

   _____

8. List four maladaptive coping mechanisms. _____

   _____

   _____

F. Closing Comments

1. Discuss the impact of the Americans with Disabilities Act Amendments Act (ADAAA) in relationship to communication barriers in healthcare.

   _____

   _____

   _____

   _____

   _____

2. Discuss three ways that healthcare providers can meet their federal obligation for accommodating patients with communication disabilities.

_____

_____

_____

CERTIFICATION PREPARATION

Circle the correct answer.

1. What is a type of nonverbal communication?
   a. Body language
   b. Oral communication
   c. Email
   d. Letter

2. What is a type of verbal communication?
   a. Written message
   b. Oral communication
   c. Email
   d. All of the above

3. Hunger, pain, anger, and tiredness are considered which type of barrier to communication?
   a. Environmental distractions
   b. Internal distractions
   c. External distractions
   d. Hearing impairment

4. What is a way to overcome environmental distractions?
   a. Help make the patient comfortable.
   b. Use audio recording and large-print materials.
   c. Provide privacy for patients.
   d. Use pictures and models.

5. What is a maladaptive coping mechanism?
   a. Passive-aggressive behavior
   b. Drug and alcohol use
   c. Denial
   d. All of the above

6. Erikson's theory places a 4-year-old child in which developmental stage?
   a. Trust versus Mistrust
   b. Autonomy versus Shame and Doubt
   c. Initiative versus Guilt
   d. Industry versus Inferiority

7. According to Kübler-Ross, when a person feels sadness, fear, and uncertainty, he is in which stage of grief?
   a. Denial
   b. Anger
   c. Bargaining
   d. Depression

8. Which level of Maslow's Hierarchy of Needs includes protection from the elements, security, and stability?
   a. Physiologic needs
   b. Safety needs
   c. Love and belongingness needs
   d. Esteem needs

9. Which level of Maslow's Hierarchy of Needs includes knowledge, curiosity, understanding, and exploration?
   a. Cognitive needs
   b. Aesthetic needs
   c. Self-actualization needs
   d. Transcendence needs

10. A person is using which defense mechanism when she reverts to an old, immature behavior to express her feelings?
   a. Denial
   b. Repression
   c. Regression
   d. Displacement

WORKPLACE APPLICATIONS

1. When Christi was doing her orientation, she observed Sally rooming patients. With the patient seated in the room, Sally stood near the patient collecting the patient's information. She smiled occasionally as she talked with the patient. Christi noticed Sally had poor posture and yawned several times during the patient interview. At times, Sally used appropriate light touch with the patient and used small hand gestures. Describe the positive nonverbal behaviors that Christi observed.

   _____

   _____

   _____

   _____

2. Using #1 above, list the negative and closed nonverbal behaviors that Christi observed. For each type of negative behavior, indicate the correct positive and open behavior that should have been used.

   _____

   _____

   _____

3. Christi is following Samantha during orientation as they work with a Hmong provider. Most of the patients are Hmong. Describe specific cultural differences with nonverbal behaviors that would apply to the Hmong community.

   _____

   _____

   _____

INTERNET ACTIVITIES

1. Using online resources, research a specific culture different than your own. Create a poster presentation, a PowerPoint presentation, or write a paper summarizing your research. Include the following points in your project:
   a. Description of the culture (e.g., origin, typical family structure)
   b. Culture, beliefs, religion, and ethnic customs that influence healthcare discussions, treatments, and care
   c. Beliefs that impact verbal and nonverbal communication

2. Using online resources, research four cultures different than your own. Focus your research on cultural beliefs that impact communication in the healthcare environment. Create a poster presentation, a PowerPoint presentation, or write a paper summarizing your research. Include tips for a medical assistant to remember when working with a patient from each of the cultures.

3. Research Maslow's Hierarchy of Needs. Create a poster presentation, a PowerPoint presentation, or write a paper summarizing the theory and describe its importance to medical assistants. Cite two appropriate references used.

4. Research adaptive (healthy) and maladaptive (nonadaptive, unhealthy) coping mechanisms. Create a list of eight adaptive and eight maladaptive coping mechanisms. Discuss the importance of using adaptive coping mechanisms. Cite two appropriate references used.

Procedure 2.1   Use Feedback Techniques and Demonstrate Respect for Individual Diversity: Gender and Appearance

Name _____ Date _____ Score _____

Tasks: Use feedback techniques (e.g., reflection, restatement, and clarification) to obtain patient information. Respond to nonverbal communication. Communicate respectfully with patients with individual diversity related to gender and appearance. Demonstrate empathy, active listening, and nonverbal communication.

Background: When working with a transgender patient, ask the patient privately which pronouns the person prefers. Make sure to add this information into the patient's health record for future reference.

Scenario: You are rooming Crystal Green. You can see that she has expertly applied her makeup, has long red fingernails, long blonde hair, and is wearing three-inch heels. You are surprised to see that her birth gender is male. This is the first time you have roomed a transgender patient. You are uncomfortable in this situation because you have strong personal beliefs that birth gender should be maintained throughout a person's life.

Directions: Role-play the scenario with a peer, who will be the patient. You need to obtain a brief medical history on this patient (e.g., chief complaint [the main reason for the visit], allergies, the pregnancy history, and the current medications). Your peer (patient) should make up any information required. Use feedback techniques to obtain her information and respond to her nonverbal communication. Demonstrate empathy, active listening, and nonverbal communication.

Equipment and Supplies:
- Patient health record
- Rooming form (optional)
- Pen

Standard: Complete the procedure and all critical steps in _____ minutes with a minimum score of 85% within two attempts (*or as indicated by the instructor*).

Scoring: Divide the points earned by the total possible points. Failure to perform a critical step, indicated by an asterisk (*), results in grade no higher than an 84% (*or as indicated by the instructor*).

Time: Began_____ Ended_____ Total minutes: _____

Steps	Possible Points	Attempt 1	Attempt 2
1. Greet the patient. Identify yourself. Verify the patient's identity with full name and date of birth. Explain the procedure in a manner that is understood by the patient. Answer any questions the patient may have on the procedure.	10		
2. Demonstrate respect for the patient. (*Refer to the Affective Behaviors Checklist – **Respect** and the Grading Rubric*)	15*		
3. Using appropriate closed and open questions and statements, obtain the patient's chief complaint (main reason for the visit), allergies, pregnancy history, and current medications. Document the information in the health record or rooming form.	10		
4. Use feedback techniques, including reflection, restatement, and clarification as information is obtained.	10*		

5.	Respond to the patient's nonverbal communication by using feedback techniques (e.g., reflection). If the patient's nonverbal communication is interpreted differently than the patient's oral statements, clarify the information with the patient.	**10***		
6.	Use active listening skills. *(Refer to the Affective Behaviors Checklist –* ***Active Listening*** *and the Grading Rubric)*	**15***		
7.	Use professional, positive nonverbal communication behaviors. *(Refer to the Affective Behaviors Checklist –* ***Nonverbal Communication*** *and the Grading Rubric)*	**15***		
8.	Demonstrate empathy by listening to the patient and learning about his or her experiences and concerns. *(Refer to the Affective Behaviors Checklist –* ***Empathy*** *and the Grading Rubric)*	**15***		
	Total Score	**100**		

Affective Behavior	**Affective Behaviors Checklist** *Directions:* Check behaviors observed during the role-play.					
Respect	**Negative, Unprofessional Behaviors**	**Attempt**		**Positive, Professional Behaviors**	**Attempt**	
		1	**2**		**1**	**2**
	Rude, unkind, fake/false attitude, disrespectful, impolite, unwelcoming			Courteous, sincere, polite, welcoming		
	Unconcerned with person's dignity; brief, abrupt			Maintained person's dignity; took time with person		
	Unprofessional verbal communication; inappropriate questions			Professional verbal communication		
	Negative nonverbal behaviors, poor eye contact			Positive nonverbal behaviors, proper eye contact		
	Other:			Other:		
Active Listening	Biased, offensive			Remained neutral		
	Interrupted			Refrained from interrupting		
	Did not allow for silence or pauses			Allowed for periods of silence		
	Negative nonverbal behaviors (rolled eyes, yawned, frowned, avoided eye contact)			Positive nonverbal behaviors (smiled, nodded head, appropriate eye contact)		
	Distracted (looked at watch, phone)			Focused on patient, avoided distractions		
	Other:			Other:		

Nonverbal Communication	Muffled voice; too fast or slow of rate; too loud or too soft; unaccepting tone			Clear voice with moderate rate and volume; varying pitch; accepting or neutral tone		
	Incorrectly pronounced words; used words the person did not understand (e.g., medical terminology, generational phrases)			Correctly pronounced words; used words person can understand		
	Stood while patient was sitting; slouching, lack of poised posture			Was at the same position of the patient; had a poised posture		
	Frowned, lack of proper eye contact, inappropriate touch			Smiled, maintained proper eye contact, used light touch on hand when appropriate		
	Other:			Other:		
Empathy	Did not listen to patient's responses			Listened to patient; learn about patient		
	Lack of respect and support demonstrated			Showed respect and support		
	Lack of therapeutic communication techniques used			Used therapeutic communication techniques		
	Negative nonverbal behaviors (e.g., positioning, frowning, poor eye contact)			Positive nonverbal behaviors (e.g., at the same level as patient, smiled, good eye contact)		
	Other:			Other:		

Grading Rubric for the Affective Behaviors Checklist *Directions: Based on checklist results, identify the points received for the procedure checklist. Indicate how the behaviors demonstrated met the expectations.*		Points for Procedure Checklist	Attempt 1	Attempt 2
Does not meet Expectation	• Response lacked respect, active listening, professional nonverbal communication, and/or empathy. • Student demonstrated more than 2 negative, unprofessional behaviors during the interaction.	0		
Needs Improvement	• Response lacked respect, active listening, professional nonverbal communication, and/or empathy. • Student demonstrated 1 or 2 negative, unprofessional behaviors during the interaction.	0		
Meets Expectation	• Response was respectful and empathetic. Demonstrated active listening, professional nonverbal communication. No negative, unprofessional behaviors observed. • More practice is needed for behavior to appear natural and for student to appear comfortable and at ease.	15		

Occasionally Exceeds Expectation	• Response was respectful and empathetic. Demonstrated active listening, professional nonverbal communication. No negative, unprofessional behaviors observed. • At times student appeared comfortable and at ease; but more practice is needed for behavior to become natural and consistent with a professional medical assistant.	15		
Always Exceeds Expectation	• Response was respectful and empathetic. Demonstrated active listening, professional nonverbal communication. No negative, unprofessional behaviors observed. • Student's behaviors appeared natural and comfortable. Behaviors are consistent with a professional medical assistant.	15		

Comments

CAAHEP Competencies	**Step(s)**
V.A.3.a. Demonstrate respect for individual diversity including: gender	2
V.A.3.f. Demonstrate respect for individual diversity including: appearance	2
V.P.1.a. Use feedback techniques to obtain patient information including: reflection	4, 5
V.P.1.b. Use feedback techniques to obtain patient information including: restatement	4
V.P.1.c. Use feedback techniques to obtain patient information including: clarification	4
V.P.2. Respond to nonverbal communication	5
V.A.1.a. Demonstrate: empathy	8
V.A.1.b. Demonstrate: active listening	6
V.A.1.c. Demonstrate: nonverbal communication	7
ABHES Competencies	**Step(s)**
5.i. Display effective interpersonal skills with patients and health care team members	Entire role-play

Procedure 2.2   Use Feedback Techniques and Demonstrate Respect for Individual Diversity: Race

Name _____ Date _____ Score _____

Tasks: Use feedback techniques (e.g., reflection, restatement, and clarification) to obtain patient information. Respond to nonverbal communication. Communicate respectfully with patients with individual diversity related to race. Demonstrate empathy, active listening, and nonverbal communication.

Background: When working with an interpreter, allow time for the person to translate the information to the patient. Also, focus on the patient and do not look at the interpreter when speaking to the patient.

Scenario: You are rooming Maria Hernandez. She is always late for her appointments, and today she was 20 minutes late. She also does not speak English and you need to use a Spanish interpreter for the visit. You are uncomfortable in this situation because you have not worked with an interpreter before. You are also feeling rushed because she was late for her appointment.

Directions: Role-play the scenario with two peers. One peer is the patient and the other peer is the interpreter. While acting as the interpreter, the information can be repeated in English. You need to obtain a brief medical history on this patient (e.g., chief complaint [the main reason for the visit], allergies, the pregnancy history, and current medications). The peer (patient) should make up any information required. Use feedback techniques to obtain her information and respond to her nonverbal communication. Demonstrate empathy, active listening, and nonverbal communication.

Equipment and Supplies:
- Patient health record
- Rooming form (optional)
- Pen

Standard: Complete the procedure and all critical steps in _____ minutes with a minimum score of 85% within two attempts (*or as indicated by the instructor*).

Scoring: Divide the points earned by the total possible points. Failure to perform a critical step, indicated by an asterisk (*), results in grade no higher than an 84% (*or as indicated by the instructor*).

Time: Began_____ Ended_____ Total minutes: _____

Steps	Possible Points	Attempt 1	Attempt 2
1. Greet the patient. Identify yourself. Verify the patient's identity with full name and date of birth. Explain the procedure in a manner that is understood by the patient. Answer any questions the patient may have on the procedure.	10		
2. Demonstrate respect for the patient. (*Refer to the Affective Behaviors Checklist – **Respect** and the Grading Rubric*)	15*		
3. Using appropriate closed and open questions and statements, obtain the patient's chief complaint (main reason for the visit), allergies, pregnancy history, and current medications. Document the information in the health record or rooming form.	10		
4. Use feedback techniques including reflection, restatements, and clarification as information is obtained.	10*		

5.	Respond to the patient's nonverbal communication by using feedback techniques (e.g., reflection). If the patient's nonverbal communication is interpreted differently than the patient's oral statements, clarify the information with the patient.	10*		
6.	Use active listening skills. *(Refer to the Affective Behaviors Checklist –* ***Active Listening*** *and the Grading Rubric)*	15*		
7.	Use professional, positive nonverbal communication behaviors. *(Refer to the Affective Behaviors Checklist –* ***Nonverbal Communication*** *and the Grading Rubric)*	15*		
8.	Demonstrate empathy by listening to the patient and learning about his or her experiences and concerns. *(Refer to the Affective Behaviors Checklist –* ***Empathy*** *and the Grading Rubric)*	15*		
	Total Score	100		

Affective Behavior	**Affective Behaviors Checklist** *Directions:* Check behaviors observed during the role-play.					
Respect	**Negative, Unprofessional Behaviors**	**Attempt**		**Positive, Professional Behaviors**	**Attempt**	
		1	**2**		**1**	**2**
	Rude, unkind, fake/false attitude, disrespectful, impolite, unwelcoming			Courteous, sincere, polite, welcoming		
	Unconcerned with person's dignity; brief, abrupt			Maintained person's dignity; took time with person		
	Focused on the interpreter; rushed the conversation; did not give the patient and interpreter time to talk			Focused on the patient; gave adequate time for the patient and interpreter to respond		
	Unprofessional verbal communication; inappropriate questions			Professional verbal communication		
	Negative nonverbal behaviors, poor eye contact			Positive nonverbal behaviors, proper eye contact		
	Other:			Other:		
Active Listening	Biased, offensive			Remained neutral		
	Interrupted			Refrained from interrupting		
	Did not allow for silence or pauses			Allowed for periods of silence		
	Negative nonverbal behaviors (rolled eyes, yawned, frowned, avoided eye contact)			Positive nonverbal behaviors, smiled, nodded head, appropriate eye contact		
	Distracted (looked at watch, phone)			Focused on patient, avoided distractions		
	Other:			Other:		

Nonverbal Communication	Muffled voice; too fast or slow of rate; too loud or too soft; unaccepting tone			Clear voice with moderate rate and volume; varying pitch; accepting or neutral tone		
	Incorrectly pronounced words; used words the person did not understand (e.g., medical terminology, generational phrases)			Correctly pronounced words; used words person can understand		
	Stood while patient was sitting; slouching, lack of poised posture			Was at the same position as the patient; had a poised posture		
	Frowned, lack of proper eye contact, inappropriate touch			Smiled, maintained proper eye contact, used light touch on hand when appropriate		
	Other:			Other:		
Empathy	Did not listen to patient's responses			Listened to patient; learned about patient		
	Lack of respect and support demonstrated			Showed respect and support		
	Lack of therapeutic communication techniques used			Used therapeutic communication techniques		
	Negative nonverbal behaviors (e.g., positioning, frowning, poor eye contact)			Positive nonverbal behaviors (e.g., at the same level as patient, smiled, good eye contact)		
	Other:			Other:		

Grading Rubric for the Affective Behaviors Checklist *Directions: Based on checklist results, identify the points received for the procedure checklist. Indicate how the behaviors demonstrated met the expectations.*		**Points for Procedure Checklist**	**Attempt 1**	**Attempt 2**
Does not meet Expectation	• Response lacked respect, active listening, professional nonverbal communication, and/or empathy. • Student demonstrated more than 2 negative, unprofessional behaviors during the interaction.	0		
Needs Improvement	• Response lacked respect, active listening, professional nonverbal communication, and/or empathy. • Student demonstrated 1 or 2 negative, unprofessional behaviors during the interaction.	0		
Meets Expectation	• Response was respectful and empathetic. Demonstrated active listening, professional nonverbal communication. No negative, unprofessional behaviors observed. • More practice is needed for behavior to appear natural and for student to appear comfortable and at ease.	15		

Occasionally Exceeds Expectation	• Response was respectful and empathetic. Demonstrated active listening, professional nonverbal communication. No negative, unprofessional behaviors observed. • At times student appeared comfortable and at ease; but more practice is needed for behavior to become natural and consistent with a professional medical assistant.	15		
Always Exceeds Expectation	• Response was respectful and empathetic. Demonstrated active listening, professional nonverbal communication. No negative, unprofessional behaviors observed. • Student's behaviors appeared natural and comfortable. Behaviors are consistent with a professional medical assistant.	15		

Comments

CAAHEP Competencies	**Step(s)**
V.A.3.b. Demonstrate respect for individual diversity including: race	2
V.A.3.f. Demonstrate respect for individual diversity including: appearance	2
V.P.1.a. Use feedback techniques to obtain patient information including: reflection	4, 5
V.P.1.b. Use feedback techniques to obtain patient information including: restatement	4
V.P.1.c. Use feedback techniques to obtain patient information including: clarification	4
V.P.2. Respond to nonverbal communication	5
V.A.1.a. Demonstrate: empathy	8
V.A.1.b. Demonstrate: active listening	6
V.A.1.c. Demonstrate: nonverbal communication	7
ABHES Competencies	**Step(s)**
5.i. Display effective interpersonal skills with patients and health care team members	Entire role-play

Procedure 2.3 Demonstrate Respect for Individual Diversity: Religion and Appearance

Name _____ Date _____ Score _____

Tasks: Respond to nonverbal communication. Communicate respectfully with patients with individual diversity related to religion and appearance. Demonstrate empathy, active listening, and nonverbal communication.

Background: The Sikh religion was founded in Northern India. Sikhs believe in one God, the equality of men and women, justice, and community service. Turbans and kachera are worn at all times for religious reasons. Turbans or scarves cover the uncut hair. If the turban or scarf needs to be removed, an alternative head covering should be provided. The turban or scarf should be treated with respect. Placing it on the floor or near shoes would be a sign of disrespect. Kachera are undershorts/undergarments and at least one leg is to remain in the kachera at all times.

Scenario: You are preparing a patient for an examination. The patient is Sikh. The provider always wants the patient to completely undress, wear a gown, and be seated on the exam table before she comes into the room. You are uncomfortable in this situation because you have never worked with a patient who is Sikh.

Directions: Role-play the scenario with a peer. Instruct the peer (patient) how to prepare for the examination. Respond to the patient's nonverbal communication. Demonstrate empathy, active listening, and nonverbal communication.

Equipment and Supplies:
- Gown and drape sheet (optional)
- Exam table (optional)

Standard: Complete the procedure and all critical steps in _____ minutes with a minimum score of 85% within two attempts (*or as indicated by the instructor*).

Scoring: Divide the points earned by the total possible points. Failure to perform a critical step, indicated by an asterisk (*), results in grade no higher than an 84% (*or as indicated by the instructor*).

Time: Began_____ Ended_____ Total minutes: _____

Steps	Possible Points	Attempt 1	Attempt 2
1. Greet the patient. Identify yourself. Verify the patient's identity with full name and date of birth. Explain the procedure (undressing) in a manner that is understood by the patient. Answer any questions the patient may have on the procedure.	20		
2. Demonstrate respect for the patient. *(Refer to the Affective Behaviors Checklist – **Respect** and the Grading Rubric)*	15*		
3. Respond to the patient's nonverbal communication by using feedback techniques (e.g., reflection). If the patient's nonverbal communication is interpreted differently than the patient's oral statements, clarify the information with the patient.	20*		
4. Use active listening skills. *(Refer to the Affective Behaviors Checklist – **Active Listening** and the Grading Rubric)*	15*		
5. Use professional, positive nonverbal communication behaviors. *(Refer to the Affective Behaviors Checklist – **Nonverbal Communication** and the Grading Rubric)*	15*		
6. Demonstrate empathy by listening to the patient and learning about his or her experiences and concerns. *(Refer to the Affective Behaviors Checklist – **Empathy** and the Grading Rubric)*	15*		
Total Score	100		

Affective Behavior	Affective Behaviors Checklist *Directions:* Check behaviors observed during the role-play.					
Respect	**Negative, Unprofessional Behaviors**	**Attempt**		**Positive, Professional Behaviors**	**Attempt**	
		1	**2**		**1**	**2**
	Rude, unkind, fake/false attitude, disrespectful, impolite, unwelcoming			Courteous, sincere, polite, welcoming		
	Unconcerned with person's dignity; brief, abrupt			Maintained person's dignity; took time with person		
	Unprofessional verbal communication; inappropriate questions			Professional verbal communication		
	Negative nonverbal behaviors, poor eye contact			Positive nonverbal behaviors, proper eye contact		
	Other:			Other:		
Active Listening	Biased, offensive			Remained neutral		
	Interrupted			Refrained from interrupting		
	Did not allow for silence or pauses			Allowed for periods of silence		
	Negative nonverbal behaviors (rolled eyes, yawned, frowned, avoided eye contact)			Positive nonverbal behaviors, smiled, nodded head, appropriate eye contact		
	Distracted (looked at watch, phone)			Focused on patient, avoided distractions		
	Other:			Other:		
Nonverbal Communication	Muffled voice; too fast or slow of rate; too loud or too soft; unaccepting tone			Clear voice with moderate rate and volume; varying pitch; accepting or neutral tone		
	Incorrectly pronounced words; used words the person did not understand (e.g., medical terminology, generational phrases)			Correctly pronounced words; used words person can understand		
	Stood while patient was sitting; slouching, lack of poised posture			Was at the same position of the patient; had a poised posture		
	Frowned. Lack of proper eye contact. Inappropriate touch.			Smiled. Maintained proper eye contact. Used light touch on hand when appropriate.		
	Other:			Other:		

Empathy	Did not listen to patient's responses			Listened to patient; learned about patient		
	Lack of respect and support demonstrated			Showed respect and support		
	Lack of therapeutic communication techniques used			Used therapeutic communication techniques		
	Negative nonverbal behaviors (e.g., positioning, frowning, poor eye contact)			Positive nonverbal behaviors (e.g., at the same level as patient, smiled, good eye contact)		
	Other:			Other:		

Grading Rubric for the Affective Behaviors Checklist ***Directions:*** *Based on checklist results, identify the points received for the procedure checklist. Indicate how the behaviors demonstrated met the expectations.*	**Points for Procedure Checklist**	**Attempt 1**	**Attempt 2**
Does not meet Expectation	• Response lacked respect, active listening, professional nonverbal communication, and/or empathy. • Student demonstrated more than 2 negative, unprofessional behaviors during the interaction.	0		
Needs Improvement	• Response lacked respect, active listening, professional nonverbal communication, and/or empathy. • Student demonstrated 1 or 2 negative, unprofessional behaviors during the interaction.	0		
Meets Expectation	• Response was respectful and empathetic. Demonstrated active listening, professional nonverbal communication. No negative, unprofessional behaviors observed. • More practice is needed for behavior to appear natural and for student to appear comfortable and at ease.	15		
Occasionally Exceeds Expectation	• Response was respectful and empathetic. Demonstrated active listening, professional nonverbal communication. No negative, unprofessional behaviors observed. • At times student appeared comfortable and at ease; but more practice is needed for behavior to become natural and consistent with a professional medical assistant.	15		
Always Exceeds Expectation	• Response was respectful and empathetic. Demonstrated active listening, professional nonverbal communication. No negative, unprofessional behaviors observed. • Student's behaviors appeared natural and comfortable. Behaviors are consistent with a professional medical assistant.	15		

Comments

CAAHEP Competencies	Step(s)
V.A.3.c. Demonstrate respect for individual diversity including: religion	2
V.A.3.f. Demonstrate respect for individual diversity including: appearance	2
V.P.2. Respond to nonverbal communication	3
V.A.1.a. Demonstrate: empathy	6
V.A.1.b. Demonstrate: active listening	4
V.A.1.c. Demonstrate: nonverbal communication	5
ABHES Competencies	**Step(s)**
5.i. Display effective interpersonal skills with patients and health care team members	Entire role-play

Procedure 2.4   Use Feedback Techniques and Demonstrate Respect for Individual Diversity: Age, Economic Status, and Appearance

Name _____ Date _____ Score _____

Tasks: Use feedback techniques (e.g., reflection, restatement, and clarification) to obtain patient information. Respond to nonverbal communication. Communicate respectfully with patients with individual diversity related to age, economic status, and appearance. Demonstrate empathy, active listening, and nonverbal communication.

Scenario: You are rooming Mr. Abraham Black (79 years old), who has recently been diagnosed with dementia. He likes to talk about things that happened long before you were born, and you are not interested in those events. He also has a hard time hearing your questions and you frequently repeat questions. Mr. Black has poor personal hygiene. His clothes are dirty and torn. He has an unpleasant body odor. Mr. Black tells you he can't afford to eat if he buys his medications. He doesn't believe in government programs and refuses to take "handouts." You have worked with Mr. Black in the past and have heard this all before numerous times. You would prefer to work with the younger generation and with patients who have better hygiene.

Directions: Role-play the scenario with a peer, who will be the patient. You need to obtain a brief medical history on this patient (e.g., chief complaint [the main reason for the visit], allergies, and the current medications). The peer (patient) should make up any information required. Use feedback techniques to obtain his information and respond to his nonverbal communication. Demonstrate empathy, active listening, and nonverbal communication.

Equipment and Supplies:
- Patient health record
- Rooming form (optional)
- Pen

Standard: Complete the procedure and all critical steps in _____ minutes with a minimum score of 85% within two attempts (*or as indicated by the instructor*).

Scoring: Divide the points earned by the total possible points. Failure to perform a critical step, indicated by an asterisk (*), results in grade no higher than an 84% (*or as indicated by the instructor*).

Time: Began_____ Ended_____ Total minutes: _____

Steps	Possible Points	Attempt 1	Attempt 2
1. Greet the patient. Identify yourself. Verify the patient's identity with full name and date of birth. Explain the procedure in a manner that is understood by the patient. Answer any questions the patient may have on the procedure.	10		
2. Demonstrate respect for the patient. (*Refer to the Affective Behaviors Checklist – **Respect** and the Grading Rubric*)	15*		
3. Using appropriate closed and open questions and statements, obtain the patient's chief complaint (main reason for the visit), allergies, and current medications. Document the information in the health record or rooming form.	10		
4. Use feedback techniques including reflection, restatement, and clarification as information is obtained.	10*		

5.	Respond to the patient's nonverbal communication by using feedback techniques (e.g., reflection). If the patient's nonverbal communication is interpreted differently than the patient's oral statements, clarify the information with the patient.	**10***		
6.	Use active listening skills. *(Refer to the Affective Behaviors Checklist – **Active Listening** and the Grading Rubric)*	**15***		
7.	Use professional, positive nonverbal communication behaviors. *(Refer to the Affective Behaviors Checklist – **Nonverbal Communication** and the Grading Rubric)*	**15***		
8.	Demonstrate empathy by listening to the patient and learning about his or her experiences and concerns. *(Refer to the Affective Behaviors Checklist – **Empathy** and the Grading Rubric)*	**15***		
	Total Score	**100**		

Affective Behavior	**Affective Behaviors Checklist** *Directions:* Check behaviors observed during the role-play.					
	Negative, Unprofessional Behaviors	**Attempt**		**Positive, Professional Behaviors**	**Attempt**	
		1	**2**		**1**	**2**
Respect	Rude, unkind, fake/false attitude, disrespectful, impolite, unwelcoming			Courteous, sincere, polite, welcoming		
	Unconcerned with person's dignity; brief, abrupt			Maintained person's dignity; took time with person		
	Unprofessional verbal communication; inappropriate questions			Professional verbal communication		
	Negative nonverbal behaviors, poor eye contact			Positive nonverbal behaviors, proper eye contact		
	Other:			Other:		
Active Listening	Biased, offensive			Remained neutral		
	Interrupted			Refrained from interrupting		
	Did not allow for silence or pauses			Allowed for periods of silence		
	Negative nonverbal behaviors (rolled eyes, yawned, frowned, avoided eye contact)			Positive nonverbal behaviors (smiled, nodded head, appropriate eye contact)		
	Distracted (looked at watch, phone)			Focused on patient, avoided distractions		
	Other:			Other:		

Nonverbal Communication	Muffled voice; too fast or slow of rate; too loud or too soft; unaccepting tone			Clear voice with moderate rate and volume; varying pitch; accepting or neutral tone		
	Incorrectly pronounced words; used words the person did not understand (e.g., medical terminology, generational phrases)			Correctly pronounced words; used words person can understand		
	Stood while patient was sitting; slouching, lack of poised posture			Was at the same position of the patient; had a poised posture		
	Frowned. Lack of proper eye contact. Inappropriate touch.			Smiled. Maintained proper eye contact. Used light touch on hand when appropriate.		
	Other:			Other:		
Empathy	Did not listen to patient's responses			Listened to patient; learned about patient		
	Lack of respect and support demonstrated			Showed respect and support		
	Lack of therapeutic communication techniques used			Used therapeutic communication techniques		
	Negative nonverbal behaviors (e.g., positioning, frowning, poor eye contact)			Positive nonverbal behaviors (e.g., at the same level as patient, smiled, good eye contact)		
	Other:			Other:		

Grading Rubric for the Affective Behaviors Checklist ***Directions:*** *Based on checklist results, identify the points received for the procedure checklist. Indicate how the behaviors demonstrated met the expectations.*		**Points for Procedure Checklist**	**Attempt 1**	**Attempt 2**
Does not meet Expectation	• Response lacked respect, active listening, professional nonverbal communication, and/or empathy. • Student demonstrated more than 2 negative, unprofessional behaviors during the interaction.	0		
Needs Improvement	• Response lacked respect, active listening, professional nonverbal communication, and/or empathy. • Student demonstrated 1 or 2 negative, unprofessional behaviors during the interaction.	0		
Meets Expectation	• Response was respectful and empathetic. Demonstrated active listening, professional nonverbal communication. No negative, unprofessional behaviors observed. • More practice is needed for behavior to appear natural and for student to appear comfortable and at ease.	15		

Occasionally Exceeds Expectation	• Response was respectful and empathetic. Demonstrated active listening, professional nonverbal communication. No negative, unprofessional behaviors observed. • At times student appeared comfortable and at ease; but more practice is needed for behavior to become natural and consistent with a professional medical assistant.	15		
Always Exceeds Expectation	• Response was respectful and empathetic. Demonstrated active listening, professional nonverbal communication. No negative, unprofessional behaviors observed. • Student's behaviors appeared natural and comfortable. Behaviors are consistent with a professional medical assistant.	15		

Comments

CAAHEP Competencies	Step(s)
V.A.3.d. Demonstrate respect for individual diversity including: age	2
V.A.3.e. Demonstrate respect for individual diversity including: economic status	2
V.A.3.f. Demonstrate respect for individual diversity including: appearance	2
V.P.1.a. Use feedback techniques to obtain patient information including: reflection	4, 5
V.P.1.b. Use feedback techniques to obtain patient information including: restatement	4
V.P.1.c. Use feedback techniques to obtain patient information including: clarification	4
V.P.2. Respond to nonverbal communication	5
V.A.1.a. Demonstrate: empathy	8
V.A.1.b. Demonstrate: active listening	6
V.A.1.c. Demonstrate: nonverbal communication	7
ABHES Competencies	**Step(s)**
5.i. Display effective interpersonal skills with patients and health care team members	Entire role-play

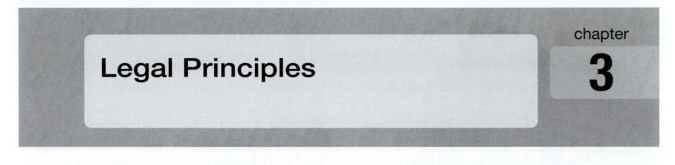

Legal Principles

chapter

3

CAAHEP Competencies	Assessment
X.C.1. Differentiate between scope of practice and standards of care for medical assistants	Skills and Concepts – G. 2
X.C.2. Compare and contrast provider and medical assistant roles in terms of standard of care	Skills and Concepts – D. 12
X.C.4. Summarize the Patient Bill of Rights	Skills and Concepts – F. 1
X.C.5. Discuss licensure and certification as they apply to healthcare providers	Skills and Concepts – G. 1 a-c
X.C.6. Compare criminal and civil law as they apply to the practicing medical assistant	Skills and Concepts – C. 2-9
X.C.7.a. Define: negligence	Vocabulary Review – G. 3; Skills and Concepts – D. 7
X.C.7.b. Define: malpractice	Vocabulary Review – G. 4; Skills and Concepts – D. 9
X.C.7.c. Define: statute of limitations	Vocabulary Review – G. 5; Certification Preparation – 2
X.C.8.a. Describe the following types of insurance: liability	Vocabulary Review – G. 11
X.C.8.b. Describe the following types of insurance: professional (malpractice)	Vocabulary Review – G. 12-13
X.C.8.c. Describe the following types of insurance: personal injury	Vocabulary Review – G. 14
X.C.13.a. Define the following medical legal terms: informed consent	Vocabulary Review – G. 20
X.C.13.b. Define the following medical legal terms: implied consent	Vocabulary Review – G. 18; Certification Preparation – 10
X.C.13.c. Define the following medical legal terms: expressed consent	Vocabulary Review – G. 19; Certification Preparation – 10
X.C.13.d. Define the following medical legal terms: patient incompetence	Vocabulary Review – G. 15
X.C.13.e. Define the following medical legal terms: emancipated minor	Vocabulary Review – G. 16
X.C.13.f. Define the following medical legal terms: mature minor	Vocabulary Review – G. 21; Certification Preparation – 8

CAAHEP Competencies	Assessment
X.C.13.g. Define the following medical legal terms: subpoena duces tecum	Vocabulary Review – G. 9; Certification Preparation – 6
X.C.13.h. Define the following medical legal terms: respondeat superior	Vocabulary Review – G. 17; Certification Preparation – 9
X.C.13.i. Define the following medical legal terms: res ipsa loquitur	Vocabulary Review – G. 10; Skills and Concepts – C. 26
X.C.13.j. Define the following medical legal terms: locum tenens	Vocabulary Review – G. 22; Certification Preparation – 7
X.C.13.k. Define the following medical legal terms: defendant-plaintiff	Vocabulary Review – G. 1-2
X.C.13.l. Define the following medical legal terms: deposition	Vocabulary Review – G. 8
X.C.13.m. Define the following medical legal terms: arbitration-mediation	Vocabulary Review – G. 6-7; Skills and Concepts – D. 21; Certification Preparation – 1
X.P.1. Locate a state's legal scope of practice for medical assistants	Procedure 3.2
X.P.4.a. Apply the Patient's Bill of Rights as it relates to: choice of treatment	Procedure 3.1
X.P.4.b. Apply the Patient's Bill of Rights as it relates to: consent for treatment	Procedure 3.1
X.P.4.c. Apply the Patient's Bill of Rights as it relates to: refusal of treatment	Procedure 3.1
X.A.1. Demonstrate sensitivity to patient rights	Procedure 3.1
ABHES Competencies	**Assessment**
4. Medical Law and Ethics c. Follow established policies when initiating or terminating medical treatment	Skills and Concepts – E. 7
4.d. Distinguish between employer and personal liability coverage	Vocabulary Review – G. 12-14 Skills and Concepts – D. 29
4.f. Comply with federal, state, and local health laws and regulations 1) Define the scope of practice for the medical assistant within the state where employed	Procedure 3.2
4.f.2) Describe what procedures can and cannot be delegated to the medical assistant and by whom within various employment settings	Skills and Concepts – G. 3 a-f

VOCABULARY REVIEW

Using the word pool on the right, find the correct word to match the definition. Write the word on the line after the definition.

Group A

1. Prone to lawsuits _____

2. A bill that has passed becomes this; also found in the name of a specific law _____

3. A rule of conduct or action prescribed or formally recognized as enforceable by a controlling authority _____

4. Used more to refer to the contents of the actual law _____

5. A piece of legislation passed by a municipality or local government _____

6. A prior court decision that serves as a model for similar legal cases in the future _____

7. Derived from legal precedents and common law _____

8. Derived from the federal and state constitutions, which gives power to federal and state governments _____

9. Unwritten laws that come from judicial decisions based on societal traditions and customs _____

10. Refers to the laws enacted by state and federal legislatures _____

Word Pool
- ordinance
- constitutional law
- statute
- litigious
- law
- common law
- precedent
- case law
- statutory law
- act

Group B

1. Laws that all parties (courts, officers, and lawyers) must follow when investigating and prosecuting unlawful acts _____

2. Laws that determine rights and obligations of people derived from common law and statutes _____

3. Lack of actions _____

4. Statutes that define actions or omissions (lack of actions) that threaten and/or harm public safety and welfare _____

5. Actions or omissions that are prohibited by criminal laws (and the government) _____

6. Protect and define private rights _____

7. A civil wrongdoing that causes harm to a person or property; excludes breach of contract _____

8. The individual or entity who committed the tort, either intentionally or as a result of negligence _____

9. Laws related to procedures, regulations, and rules of governmental administrative agencies _____

10. A monetary settlement the defendant pays the plaintiff in a civil case for loss or injury _____

Word Pool
- tort
- damages
- criminal law
- regulatory and administrative law
- civil laws
- procedural law
- tortfeasor
- crimes
- substantive law
- omissions

Group C

1. A court order by which an individual or institution is required to perform or refrain from performing a certain act

   _____

2. Applies reasonable behavior as an objective test to measure another's actions or lack of actions _____

3. A court judgment that defines the legal rights of the parties involved _____

4. Refers to the level and type of care an ordinary, prudent healthcare professional having the same training and experience in a similar practice would have provided under a similar situation _____

5. Range of responsibilities and practice guidelines that determine the boundaries within which a healthcare worker practices

   _____

6. A strategy used by the defendant to avoid liability in a lawsuit

   _____

7. Latin for "a thing decided;" once a case has been decided by the court, it cannot be litigated again _____

8. The process of settling disputes outside of litigation

   _____

9. A legal obligation _____

10. A process that can be used if there are no disputes about the facts in the case _____

Word Pool
- declaratory judgment
- standard of care
- scope of practice
- injunction
- alternative dispute resolution
- reasonable person standard
- *res judicata*
- defense
- summary judgment
- legally binding

Group D

1. A court order requiring a person to appear in court at a specific time to testify in a legal case _____

2. Written or oral questions that must be answered under oath

   _____

3. People who observed the situation and testify in court about the facts of the case _____

4. People who are educated and knowledgeable in the area of concern; the testify in court and provide an expert opinion on the topic of concern _____

5. A settlement for a specific dollar amount that directly relates to medical bills _____

6. Very large payment meant to punish the defendant

   _____

7. A settlement for losses suffered; losses can be related to loss of income, property damage, and medical care

   _____

8. The person or company purchasing the insurance policy

   _____

9. Very small settlement because the plaintiff's injury was slight

   _____

10. A settlement for emotional pain and anguish, loss of future earning power, and so on _____

Word Pool
- special damages
- general damages
- nominal damages
- expert witnesses
- subpoena
- compensatory damages
- punitive damages
- interrogatory
- insured
- fact witnesses

Group E

1. Legally responsible or obligated _____
2. The payment the insured pays to the insurance company _____
3. Another name for the insurance company _____
4. When the insurer pays the plaintiff, the plaintiff is known as the _____
5. An agreement between two parties _____
6. The parties have agreed to the terms of the contract through their actions and behaviors _____
7. A form of medical malpractice, also called *negligent termination*; the provider ends the provider-patient relationship without reasonable or adequate notification _____
8. The parties have specifically stated the terms of the contract in writing, orally, or both _____
9. One who has not reached adulthood; usually age 18 or 21 depending on the jurisdiction _____
10. Occurs when the terms of the contract are not fulfilled by one party without a legitimate legal reason _____

Word Pool
- implied contract
- patient abandonment
- insurer
- contract
- premium
- third party
- minor
- liable
- expressed contract
- breach of contract

Group F

1. One party voluntarily agrees with another party's proposition or plan _____
2. A mandatory process established by state law that ensures a person has met the legal standards for practicing an occupation in that state _____
3. A voluntary process indicating that a person has met predetermined criteria _____
4. The use of telecommunication technology to provide healthcare services to patients at a distance; it is usually used in rural communities _____
5. License is terminated and the person can no longer practice in that occupation in the state _____
6. Person's license is monitored for a specific period of time _____
7. Person cannot practice in that occupation for a specific period of time _____
8. Person is sent a warning or letter of concern _____
9. Person voluntarily gives up license _____
10. Recognition granted by a specific organization to educational, healthcare, or managed care organizations that have demonstrated compliance with standards _____

Word Pool
- telemedicine
- license surrendered
- probation
- consent
- accreditation
- certification
- reprimand
- license revoked
- license suspended
- licensure

Group G

Define each word or phrase.

1. Plaintiff: _____

_____

2. Defendant: _____

_____

3. Negligence: _____

_____

4. Malpractice: _____

_____

5. Statute of limitation: _____

_____

6. Arbitration: _____

_____

7. Mediation: _____

_____

8. Deposition: _____

_____

9. *Subpoena duces tecum*: _____

_____

10. *Res ipsa loquitur*: _____

_____

11. Liability insurance: _____

_____

12. Professional liability insurance: _____

_____

13. Medical malpractice insurance: _____

_____

14. Personal injury insurance: _____

_____

15. (Patient) incompetence: _____

_____

16. Emancipated minor: _____

_____

17. *Respondeat superior*: _____

_____

18. Implied consent: _____

_____

19. Expressed consent: _____

_____

20. Informed consent: _____

_____

21. Mature minor: _____

_____

22. *Locum tenens*: _____

_____

ABBREVIATIONS
Write out what each of the following abbreviations stands for.

1. DOB: _____

2. VIS: _____

3. CMA: _____

4. LPN: _____

5. NP: _____

6. CNM: _____

7. RN: _____

8. PA: _____

9. MD: _____

10. DO: _____

11. OWI: _____

12. OUI: _____

13. ADR: _____

14. CDC: _____

15. CAAHEP: _____

SKILLS AND CONCEPTS
Answer the following questions. Write your answer on the line or in the space provided.

A. Introduction to Law

1. Why is it important for medical assistants to learn about law?_____

_____

_____

B. Sources of Law

1. A(n) _____ is a rule of conduct or action prescribed or formally recognized as enforceable by a controlling authority.

2. The _____ is the supreme law of the United States.

3. The _____ branch includes the Supreme Court and interprets laws according to the U.S. Constitution.

4. The _____ branch includes Congress and makes new laws.

5. The president administers the _____ branch and issues executive orders, appoints judges, and makes treaties with other nations.

6. Case law was derived from legal _____ and _____.

C. Criminal and Civil Law

1. _____ law determines the rights and obligations of the people and _____ laws must be followed when investigating and prosecuting unlawful acts.

2. When criminal cases are brought to court, the _____ is the government and the _____ is the person or party charged with the offense.

3. With civil law, the _____ is the victim of the wrongdoing and the _____ is the wrongdoer.

4. In criminal law, the wrongdoing is called a(n) _____ and in civil law it can be called a(n) _____ or a(n) _____.

5. A(n) _____, a serious criminal offense, is punishable by a substantial fine and _____ time _____ 1 year.

6. A(n) _____, a lesser criminal offense, is punishable by a substantial fine and possible _____ time _____ 1 year.

7. Name five common types of disputes handled in the civil court system. _____

_____

8. If the matter is brought to court, in the _____ court system, most of the time there is a trial by jury; whereas with the _____ court system, cases are decided by the judge and many times there is no jury.

9. Compare criminal and civil law as they apply to the practicing medical assistant. Your answer should also provide an example of a criminal and civil matter that relates to medical assistants. (Provide examples other than those in the textbook.)

_____

_____

_____

_____

_____

D. Tort Law

1. Describe the two types of torts discussed in the textbook. _____

_____

_____

_____

2. _____ is disclosing private facts without the consent of the individual or intrusion into a person's personal life.

3. _____ is the intentional restraint of another individual without consent or reason.

4. _____ is deceiving or lying to a person or party for monetary gain.

5. _____ is intentionally saying something or writing something false about another person that causes harm.

6. _____ is written defamation and _____ is spoken defamation.

7. Explain the "reasonable person" standard and how it can determine negligent acts. _____

_____

_____

8. Describe the negligent acts of malfeasance, misfeasance, and nonfeasance. _____

_____

_____

_____

_____

9. Describe when medical malpractice occurs. _____

   _____

   _____

10. How does medical malpractice differ from negligence?_____

    _____

    _____

11. Describe "standard of care." _____

    _____

    _____

12. Discuss how the provider's and the medical assistant's roles are similar and yet different in terms of standard of care.

    _____

    _____

    _____

13. Name the three main types of defenses. _____

    _____

14. _____, a technical defense that varies by state, gives the length of time legal action can be taken after an event has occurred.

15. List the three requirements for Good Samaritan protection. _____

    _____

    _____

16. Describe *res judicata* and how it is used as a technical defense._____

    _____

    _____

17. What defense is used when none of the facts are true?_____

18. Describe affirmative defense. _____

    _____

    _____

19. _____ is an affirmative defense, which means the plaintiff's action or lack of action caused the injury to a certain percent.

20. _____ is an affirmative defense, which means the defendant can show evidence that the plaintiff knew about the risks involved and consented to proceed with the activity.

21. Describe the two types of alternative dispute resolution. _____

_____

_____

22. What is a summary judgment and why is it used? _____

_____

_____

23. Describe the four "Ds" or four elements that must be proven in malpractice cases. _____

_____

_____

_____

24. Briefly describe the stages of a civil lawsuit. _____

_____

_____

_____

25. Discuss the difference between an expert witness and a fact witness. _____

_____

_____

_____

26. Describe *res ipsa loquitur* and when it is used. _____

_____

_____

_____

27. _____ are large payments made to the plaintiff by the defendant, meant to punish the defendant.

28. _____ are a monetary payment for losses suffered.

29. Describe general liability or commercial liability insurance. _____

_____

_____

30. _____ are monetary payments for emotional pain and anguish.

31. A(n) _____ covers for claims that are made during the policy year, whereas _____ covers claims for lawful acts that occurred during the policy year.

E. Contracts

1. Describe the difference between implied contracts and expressed contracts._____

    _____

2. Describe the statute of frauds and give three types of contracts to which it applies. _____

    _____

    _____

3. Describe the five elements required for a legally binding contract. _____

    _____

    _____

    _____

4. Name three conditions related to competency and capacity that would invalidate a contract._____

    _____

5. Name four benefits of becoming an emancipated minor. _____

    _____

    _____

6. List three reasons providers terminate the provider-patient relationship. _____

    _____

    _____

7. Describe the process of terminating the provider-patient relationship._____

    _____

    _____

    _____

8. Providers can be charged with _____ if they do not follow the proper termination procedure.

9. How can a medical assistant protect the provider from charges of patient abandonment?_____

    _____

    _____

10. List three ways breach of contract can occur in healthcare. _____

    _____

    _____

    _____

11. List the seven elements that must be present for informed consent. _____

_____

_____

_____

12. List five types of patients who can give informed consent. _____

_____

_____

13. List four types of patients who cannot give informed consent._____

_____

_____

14. Describe the medical assistant's role in informed consent. _____

_____

_____

F. Patient's Bill of Rights

1. Summarize the Patient's Bill of Rights. _____

_____

_____

_____

_____

2. A patient refuses an injection of medication ordered by the provider. Describe the steps that need to be followed by the medical assistant.

_____

_____

_____

_____

G. Practice Requirements

1. Describe the licensure and certification for the following healthcare professionals:

    a. Doctor of medicine (MD) and doctor of osteopathy (DO): _____

    _____

b. Physician assistant (PA):_____

_____

c. Nurse practitioner (NP): _____

_____

d. Medical assistant (MA): _____

_____

e. Registered nurse (RN) and licensed practical nurse (LPN): _____

_____

2. Differentiate between the scope of practice and standard of care for medical assistants._____

_____

_____

_____

3. For the following activities, identify if the medical assistant could be delegated (assigned) by the provider to do the activity. Write "yes" on the line if the medical assistant could be delegated the activity. Write "no" on the line if the medical assistant could not do the activity.

a. Prepare the informed consent paperwork. _____

b. Discuss the procedure with the patient for the informed consent. _____

c. Prepare waived laboratory testing. _____

d. Answer phone calls. _____

e. Prescribe medications for the patient's condition. _____

f. Diagnose the patient's condition. _____

CERTIFICATION PREPARATION
Circle the correct answer.

1. Which is a type of alternative dispute resolution where the final decision is legally binding?
    a. Dereliction
    b. Mediation
    c. Arbitration
    d. Summary judgment

2. Which varies by state and indicates the length of time legal action can be taken after an event has occurred?
    a. *Res judicata*
    b. *Res ipsa loquitur*
    c. Release of tortfeasor
    d. Statute of limitations

3. Which is a negligent act classification that means the person failed to act when he or she had a legal duty to act?
    a. Misfeasance
    b. Nonfeasance
    c. Malpractice
    d. Malfeasance

4. Which type of defense involves the defendant admitting wrongdoing and the defense attorney introduces facts that support the defendant's conduct?
    a. Denial defense
    b. Comparative defense
    c. Technical defense
    d. Affirmative defense

5. Which is not one of the "Ds" of negligence?
   a. Duty of care
   b. Dereliction
   c. Deposition
   d. Damages

6. Which is a legal document ordering a person to bring the plaintiff's health record to court?
   a. Subpoena
   b. *Subpoena duces tecum*
   c. *Res ipsa loquitur*
   d. Statute of limitations

7. Which is a physician or advanced-practice professional temporarily contracted to provide healthcare services when a facility has a vacancy, vacation, or a leave of absence?
   a. Telemedicine
   b. Injunction
   c. *Respondeat superior*
   d. *Locum tenens*

8. A person younger than the age of adulthood who demonstrates the maturity to make a personal healthcare decision and can give informed consent for treatment is called a(n)
   a. mature minor.
   b. emancipated minor.
   c. incompetence.
   d. *respondeat superior.*

9. Which means "let the master answer;" thus, the employer/provider is legally responsible for the wrongful actions or lack of actions of the employees if done within the scope of employment?
   a. Tortfeasor
   b. *Res ipsa loquitur*
   c. *Respondeat superior*
   d. *Res judicata*

10. _____ consent is inferred based on signs or conduct of the patient, whereas _____ is given either by the spoken or written word.
    a. Implied; informed
    b. Informed; expressed
    c. Implied; expressed
    d. Expressed; informed

WORKPLACE APPLICATIONS

1. Cara was just graduating from a medical assistant program and decided to take out a professional liability insurance policy. She wants a policy that she can stop paying at retirement and will still be covered for past situations. Describe what type of policy she should purchase.

   _____

   _____

   _____

   _____

2. Dr. Smith and Dr. Brown are family practice providers who trained at the same college. Dr. Smith practices in Los Angeles, CA and Dr. Brown practices in Bayfield, WI (a city of 475 people). Would the standard of care be the same for these two family practice providers? Explain your answer.

   _____

   _____

   _____

3. Jane is a medical assistant who works with Dr. Walden. She identifies herself as "Dr. Walden's nurse" to patients. Discuss how this might impact the standard of care.

   _____

   _____

4. Ken Thomas was notified by a medical supplier that the mesh that was used for his hernia surgery was faulty. They paid Ken a monetary compensation after Ken signed a release to give up the right to sue the company in the future. Five years later, Ken had to go through surgery to remove the mesh. Ken wanted to sue the company for his pain and suffering. What technical defense would be used to prevent the lawsuit? Discuss this technical defense.

   _____

   _____

   _____

5. Bella, a new CMA, is working with a patient who is undergoing minor surgery. The provider explained the procedure and stepped out of the room. She needs to get the informed consent form signed. When she asks the patient if she has any questions before signing, the patient states she does. How should Bella handle this situation?

   _____

   _____

   _____

INTERNET ACTIVITIES

1. Using the internet, find a local healthcare facility that has their Patient's Bill of Rights posted online. Create a poster presentation or a PowerPoint presentation summarizing the areas addressed in the facility's Patient's Bill of Rights.

2. Using online resources, research how an MD and/or DO can renew his or her license in your state. Write a brief summary of what is required to renew a medical doctor's license in your state. Cite the website(s) used.

3. Credentialed medical assistants need to maintain their credentials through continuing education. Using online resources, identify two sites that offer continuing education for medical assistants. Briefly summarize your findings and cite the websites used.

Procedure 3.1   Apply the Patient's Bill of Rights

Name _____   Date _____   Score _____

Tasks: Apply the patient's bill of rights in scenarios related to choice of treatment, consent for treatment, and refusal of treatment. Demonstrate sensitivity to patient rights.

Scenario 1 (Choice of treatment): Julia Berkley (DOB 7/5/1992) was a patient of Dr. Angela Perez during her entire pregnancy. Julia is experiencing some complications. Dr. Perez explained the choices Julia had for delivery. She stated with the complications, a C-section may be the best option. You are working with Dr. Perez and prepared the consent form for the C-section. You go into the exam room to have Julia sign the consent form. As you discuss the form, Julia tells you that she is fearful of a C-section and wants a vaginal delivery.

Scenario 2 (Consent for treatment): Ken Thomas (DOB 10/25/61) saw Jean Burke N.P. before leaving on a week-long trip out of the country. He is leaving in 3 days and wants a hepatitis A vaccine injection. The area he is traveling to has a high risk for hepatitis A. Jean Burke orders immunoglobulin for Ken, which will provide immediate protection against hepatitis A. You prepare the injection and enter the exam room. As you are telling Ken about the side effects of the medication, he asks, "What is immunoglobulin?" You reply that it is a sterile medication made of antibodies from blood. Ken states that he is a Jehovah's Witness and cannot receive blood products.

Scenario 3 (Refusal of treatment): Aaron Jackson (DOB 10/17/2011) was in for his well-child check. His records indicate that he is due for his first varicella vaccine. You bring the Varicella (Chickenpox) Vaccine VIS (vaccine information statement) and the Vaccine Authorization form to the exam room. As you start discussing the vaccine, Aaron's mother, Patricia, interrupts you and tells you she is not interested in having Aaron get his chickenpox vaccine.

Equipment and Supplies:
- Patient health records
- Patient's Bill of Rights (Figure 3.3)
- General Procedure Consent form (Figure 3.4)
- Varicella (Chickenpox) VIS (available at www.cdc.gov)
- Vaccine Authorization form (Figure 3.5)

Standard: Complete the procedure and all critical steps in _____ minutes with a minimum score of 85% within two attempts (*or as indicated by the instructor*).

Scoring: Divide the points earned by the total possible points. Failure to perform a critical step, indicated by an asterisk (*), results in grade no higher than an 84% (*or as indicated by the instructor*).

Time: Began_____ Ended_____ Total minutes: _____

Steps:	Point Value	Attempt 1	Attempt 2
1. Review the Patient's Bill of Rights. Apply the Patient's Bill of Rights as you role-play each of the three scenarios.	10*		
2. Using Scenario #1, role-play the situation with a peer. You are the medical assistant. Demonstrate how a medical assistant should handle the situation. Apply the Patient's Bill of Rights to the situation by remembering the rights of the patient. a. Show sensitivity to the patient by being respective and professional. *(Refer to the Checklist for Affective Behaviors.)*	10*		
b. Ask the patient if she has any questions about the procedures. Let the provider know if the patient has questions.	10		
c. Ask the patient what she would like to do. Based on her answer, follow up as necessary.	10*		
d. Using the health record, document the patient's decision and the name of the provider notified.	5		
3. Using Scenario #2, role-play the situation with a peer. You are the medical assistant. Demonstrate how a medical assistant should handle the situation. Apply the Patient's Bill of Rights to the situation by remembering the rights of the patient. a. Show sensitivity to the patient regarding his right to refuse. Be accepting of his beliefs and his refusal. *(Refer to the Checklist for Affective Behaviors.)*	10*		
b. When the patient refuses the medication, be respectful in your body language and words. Notify the provider.	10*		
c. Using the health record, document the patient's decision and the name of the provider notified.	5		
4. Using Scenario #3, role-play the situation with a peer. You are the medical assistant. Demonstrate how a medical assistant should handle the situation. Apply the Patient's Bill of Rights to the situation by remembering the rights of the patient. a. Show sensitivity to the mother of the patient by being respectful and professional. *(Refer to the Checklist for Affective Behaviors.)*	10*		
b. Ask the mother if she has any questions about the vaccine. Let the provider know if the mother has questions.	5		
c. Ask the mother what she would like to do. Based on her answer, follow up as necessary.	10*		
d. Using the health record, document the mother's decision and the name of the provider notified.	5		
Total Points	100		

Checklist for Affective Behaviors

Affective Behavior	Directions: Check behaviors observed during the role-play.				
Sensitivity	**Negative, Unprofessional Behaviors**	**Attempt 1**	**Attempt 2**	**Positive, Professional Behaviors**	**Attempt 1**	**Attempt 2**
	Poor eye contact			Proper eye contact		
	Distracted; not focused on the other person			Focuses full attention on the other person		
	Judgmental attitude; not accepting attitude			Nonjudgmental, accepting attitude		
	Fails to clarify what the person verbally or nonverbally communicated			Uses summarizing or paraphrasing to clarify what the person verbally or nonverbally communicated		
	Fails to acknowledge what the person communicated			Acknowledges what the person communicated		
	Rude, discourteous			Pleasant and courteous		
	Disregards the person's dignity and rights			Maintains the person's dignity and rights		
	Other:			Other:		

Grading for Affective Behaviors		Point Value	Attempt 1	Attempt 2
Does not meet Expectation	• Response lacked sensitivity. • Student demonstrated more than 2 negative, unprofessional behaviors during the interaction.	0		
Needs Improvement	• Response lacked sensitivity. • Student demonstrated 1 or 2 negative, unprofessional behaviors during the interaction.	0		
Meets Expectation	• Response was sensitive; no negative, unprofessional behaviors observed. • More practice is needed for behavior to appear natural and for student to appear comfortable and at ease.	10		
Occasionally Exceeds Expectation	• Response was sensitive; no negative, unprofessional behaviors observed. • At times student appeared comfortable and at ease; but more practice is needed for behavior to become natural and consistent with a professional medical assistant.	10		
Always Exceeds Expectation	• Response was sensitive; no negative, unprofessional behaviors observed. • Student's behaviors appeared natural and comfortable. Behaviors are consistent with a professional medical assistant.	10		

Documentation – Scenario 1

Documentation – Scenario 2

Documentation – Scenario 3

Comments

CAAHEP Competencies	Steps
X.P.4.a. Apply the Patient's Bill of Rights as it relates to: choice of treatment	1, 2 a-d
X.P.4.b. Apply the Patient's Bill of Rights as it relates to: consent for treatment	1, 3 a-c
X.P.4.c. Apply the Patient's Bill of Rights as it relates to: refusal of treatment	1, 4 a-d
X.A.1. Demonstrate sensitivity to patient rights	2 a, 3 a, 4 a

Procedure 3.2   Locate the Medical Assistant's Legal Scope of Practice

Name _____ Date _____ Score _____

Tasks: Locate the legal scope of practice for a medical assistant practicing in your state. Summarize the scope of practice.

Equipment and Supplies:
- Computer and printer with word processing software and internet access

Standard: Complete the procedure and all critical steps with a minimum score of 85% within two attempts (*or as indicated by the instructor*).

Scoring: Divide the points earned by the total possible points. Failure to perform a critical step, indicated by an asterisk (*), results in grade no higher than an 84% (*or as indicated by the instructor*).

Steps:	Point Value	Attempt 1	Attempt 2
1. Using the internet, search for the medical assistant's scope of practice in your state. Read the scope of practice for your state.	20		
2. Using the word processing software, create a short paper summarizing the medical assistant's scope of practice. Address the following points: a. Can medical assistants give injections? If so, what type of injections? b. Can medical assistants give oral, topical, and/or inhaled medications? c. Can medical assistants calculate drug dosages? d. What is the medical assistant's role with prescriptions? e. Describe additional duties that a medical assistant can legally do in your state. f. Include the website address(es) you used for this paper. *Note:* If your instructor does not provide you with different guidelines for the paper, follow these. Create at least a one-page paper, using double line spacing and a 10-12 point font. Margins should be 1" for all sides.	70		
3. After completing the paper, proofread it. Use correct spelling, punctuation, sentence structure, and capitalization. Make any changes required. Based on your instructor's directions, submit the paper to the instructor.	10		
Total Points	100		

Comments

CAAHEP Competencies	Step(s)
X.P.1. Locate a state's legal scope of practice for medical assistants	Entire procedure
ABHES Competencies	**Step(s)**
4.f.1 Define the scope of practice for the medical assistant within the state where employed	Entire procedure

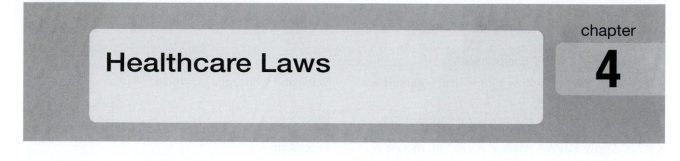

chapter

Healthcare Laws

4

CAAHEP Competencies	Assessment
X.C.3. Describe components of the Health Information Portability & Accountability Act (HIPAA)	Skills and Concepts – B. 2-7, 13-14; Certification Preparation – 4-7; Workplace Application 1 a-d, 2-3
X.C.7.d. Define: Good Samaritan Act(s)	Skills and Concepts – C. 16-18; Certification Preparation – 1
X.C.7.e. Define: Uniform Anatomical Gift Act	Skills and Concepts – C. 21; Certification Preparation – 2
X.C.7.h. Define: Patient Self Determination Act (PSDA)	Skills and Concepts – C. 19; Certification Preparation – 1
X.C.7.i. Define: risk management	Skills and Concepts – D. 28
X.C.9. List and discuss legal and illegal applicant interview questions	Skills and Concepts – D. 20-22; Certification Preparation – 9
X.C.10.a. Identify: Health Information Technology for Economic and Clinical Health (HITECH) Act	Skills and Concepts – B. 15-17
X.C.10.b. Identify: Genetic Information Nondiscrimination Act of 2008 (GINA)	Skills and Concepts – B. 18-19, D. 19
X.C.10.c. Identify: Americans with Disabilities Act Amendments Act (ADAAA)	Skills and Concepts – D. 23; Certification Preparation – 10
X.C.11.a. Describe the process in compliance reporting: unsafe activities	Skills and Concepts – D. 24
X.C.11.b. Describe the process in compliance reporting: errors in patient care	Skills and Concepts – D. 29
X.C.11.c. Describe the process in compliance reporting: conflicts of interest	Skills and Concepts – D. 11-12
X.C.11.d. Describe the process in compliance reporting: incident reports	Skills and Concepts – D. 25-27
X.C.12.a. Describe compliance with public health statutes: communicable diseases	Skills and Concepts – D. 2 a-d
X.C.12.b. Describe compliance with public health statutes: abuse, neglect, and exploitation	Skills and Concepts – D. 5-7; Workplace Application – 4
X.C.12.c. Describe compliance with public health statutes: wounds of violence	Skills and Concepts – D. 3-4

CAAHEP Competencies	Assessment
X.C.13.n. Define the following medical legal terms: Good Samaritan laws	Skills and Concepts – C. 16-18
X.P.2.a. Apply HIPAA rules in regard to: privacy	Procedure 4.1
X.P.2.b. Apply HIPAA rules in regard to: release of information	Procedure 4.2
X.P.5. Perform compliance reporting based on public health statutes	Procedure 4.3
X.P.6. Report an illegal activity in the healthcare setting following proper protocol	Procedure 4.4
X.P.7. Complete an incident report related to an error in patient care	Procedure 4.5
X.A.1. Demonstrate sensitivity to patient rights	Procedure 4.1

ABHES Competencies	Assessment
4. Medical Law and Ethics b. Institute federal and state guidelines when: 1) Releasing medical records or information	Procedure 4.1, 4.2
4.b.2) Entering orders in and utilizing electronic health records	Procedure 4.3
4.e. Perform risk management procedures	Procedure 4.5
4.f. Comply with federal, state, and local health laws and regulations as they relate to healthcare settings	Procedure 4.1, 4.2, 4.3, 4.4
4.h. Demonstrate compliance with HIPAA guidelines, the ADA Amendments Act, and the Health Information Technology for Economic and Clinical Health (HITECH) Act	Procedure 4.1, 4.2

VOCABULARY REVIEW

Using the word pool on the right, find the correct word to match the definition. Write the word on the line after the definition.

Group A

1. Step-by-step directions _____
2. The electronic exchange of information between two agencies to accomplish financial or administrative healthcare activities _____
3. An organization that accepts the claim data from the provider, reformats the data to meet the specifications outlined by the insurance plan, and submits the claim _____
4. A system designed to use characters (i.e., numbers and letters) to represent something like a medical procedure or a disease _____
5. Written principles that provide goals for the employees and the facility _____
6. Being free from unwanted intrusion _____
7. The top priority _____
8. A legally protected right of patients _____
9. The disclosing of private facts without the consent of the individual _____
10. Conforms to nationally recognized standards and contains health-related information about a specific patient; it can be created, managed, and consulted by authorized clinicians and staff from more than one healthcare organization _____

Word Pool
- privacy
- claims clearinghouse
- confidentiality
- coding system
- electronic health record
- invasion of privacy
- precedence
- policies
- procedures
- electronic transaction

Group B

1. Individually identifiable health information stored or transmitted by covered entities or business associates _____

2. Protected health information that has had all of the direct patient identifiers removed _____

3. Reasons that the health information can be released _____

4. Healthcare providers, health (insurance) plans, and claims clearinghouses that transmit protected health information electronically _____

5. A form that must be completed by the patient before information can be shared with another person; also called an *authorization to disclose form* _____

6. To remove all direct patient identifiers from the PHI information _____

7. A form that must be completed by the patient before the patient records can be transferred _____

8. A person or business that provides a service to a covered entity that involves access to PHI _____

9. Safeguards that include a security officer who is responsible _____

10. Safeguards that include facility, workstation, and device security _____

Word Pool
- covered entities
- business associate
- permission
- administrative safeguards
- physical safeguards
- protected health information
- record release form
- de-identify
- limited data set
- disclosure authorization

Group C

1. Disclosure of protected health information, without a reason or permission, which compromises the security or privacy of the information _____

2. Leaving a place; exit route _____

3. Diseases spread from person to person by either direct contact or indirect contact _____

4. An action that purposely harms another person _____

5. Written instructions about healthcare decisions in case a person is unable to make them _____

6. Failure to provide proper attention or care to another person _____

7. The act of using another person for one's own advantage _____

8. Communication that cannot be disclosed without authorization of the person involved; includes provider-patient and lawyer-client communications _____

9. People between the ages of 18 and 64 who have a mental or physical impairment that prevents them from doing normal activities or from protecting themselves _____

10. Getting back at others for something they did to you _____

Word Pool
- egress
- abuse
- advance directives
- retaliation
- breach
- communicable diseases
- dependent adults
- privileged communication
- exploitation
- neglect

Group D

1. Any financial interest, personal or professional activity, or obligation that impacts a person's objectivity when performing the job _____

2. Punishment inflicted on someone as vengeance for a wrong or criminal act; the act of taking revenge _____

3. A deceitful action that causes another to give up something of value _____

4. The employer can end employment at any time for any reason _____

5. Legal reason for firing an employee _____

6. Employer did not have just cause for firing the employee _____

7. Unfair treatment of another person based on the person's age, gender (sex), ethnicity, sexual orientation, disability, marital status, or other selective factors _____

8. Continued, unwanted, and annoying actions done to another person _____

9. A person (usually an employee) who reports a violation of the law within the organization; the person reports the information to the public or to a person in authority _____

Word Pool
- fraud
- retribution
- conflict of interest
- wrongful termination
- just cause
- harassment
- employment-at-will
- discrimination
- whistleblower

ABBREVIATIONS
Write out what each of the following abbreviations stands for.

1. HIPAA _____
2. EHR _____
3. HHS _____
4. OCR _____
5. CPT _____
6. ICD _____
7. NPI _____
8. HPI _____
9. EIN _____
10. PHI _____
11. ePHI _____
12. FDA _____
13. DEA _____
14. PPSA _____

15. CMS _____

16. CLIA _____

17. OSH Act _____

18. OSHA _____

19. OPIM _____

20. PPE _____

21. CAPTA _____

22. VAERS _____

23. CDC _____

24. VICP _____

25. UDDA _____

26. UAGA _____

27. NOTA _____

28. OPTN _____

SKILLS AND CONCEPTS

Answer the following questions. Write your answer on the line or in the space provided.

A. Privacy and Confidentiality

1. Describe privacy and an invasion of privacy. _____

   _____

   _____

   _____

2. Healthcare professionals have a duty to maintain the confidentiality of patients. Describe what this means in your own words.

   _____

   _____

   _____

3. If your state's confidentiality laws are stricter than the federal laws, the state laws need to be followed. This is known as _____.

B. Health Insurance Portability and Accountability Act

1. The _____ enforces HIPAA.

2. Describe the following components of HIPAA.

   a. Standard 1 related to transactions and code sets: _____

   _____

   _____

   b. Standard 2 related to the Privacy Rule: _____

   _____

   _____

   c. Standard 3 related to the Security Rule: _____

   _____

   _____

   d. Standard 4 related to unique identifiers: _____

   _____

   _____

3. List five covered entities. _____

   _____

   _____

4. Define *business associates* and give two examples. _____

   _____

   _____

   _____

5. What is the main purpose of the Privacy Rule? _____

   _____

6. Patients have rights over their information. List three of these rights. _____

   _____

   _____

7. List six permissions that do not require written patient authorization. _____

   _____

   _____

   _____

8. When patients are being treated for emotional or mental conditions, the _____ allows providers to use professional judgment to determine if the records should be released to the patients.

9. List three parts of a patient record that are held at a higher level of confidentiality. _____

   _____

   _____

10. Describe what psychotherapy notes include. _____

    _____

    _____

11. To maintain higher levels of confidentiality with psychotherapy notes, explain strategies used to limit access to these notes.

    _____

    _____

12. Briefly describe the Alcohol and Drug Abuse Patient Records Privacy Law. _____

    _____

    _____

13. The _____ covers patient records that are created, used, received, and maintained by the covered entities.

14. Describe physical and technical safeguards that are used to ensure the security of the ePHI. _____

    _____

    _____

    _____

    _____

15. What does HITECH stand for? _____

    _____

16. What provisions were included in the HITECH Act? _____

    _____

    _____

17. Describe how the HITECH Act modified HIPAA. _____

    _____

    _____

    _____

    _____

18. What does GINA stand for? _____

19. Describe the importance of GINA. _____

_____

_____

C. Additional Healthcare Laws and Regulations

1. The _____ enforces the Food, Drug, and Cosmetic Act.

2. Describe what the FDA is responsible for. _____

_____

3. Name five areas overseen by the FDA. _____

_____

4. The _____ enforces the Controlled Substances Act.

5. List the areas overseen by the DEA. _____

_____

6. Schedule _____ has the highest potential for abuse and Schedule _____ has the lowest potential for abuse.

7. Each provider prescribing scheduled medications needs to have a unique _____ that needs to be renewed every _____.

8. The _____ is commonly known as the Affordable Care Act.

9. What was the goal of the Affordable Care Act? _____

_____

10. Describe the purpose of Physician Payments Sunshine Act. _____

_____

_____

11. _____ establishes quality standards and regulates laboratory testing.

12. Occupational Safety and Health Act of 1970 is enforced by the _____.

13. List two things that the Occupational Safety and Health Administration does based on the Occupational Safety and Health Act.

_____

_____

14. What is the goal of the Needlestick Safety and Prevention Act? _____

_____

15. What is the Needlestick Safety and Prevention Act's impact on healthcare workers? _____

_____

_____

16. Describe the Good Samaritan laws (or acts). _____

_____

17. List the three requirements the person responding to the emergency must meet under the Good Samaritan law (or act).

_____

_____

_____

18. Why is it important for healthcare workers to know their state's Good Samaritan law? _____

_____

19. Describe the Patient Self-Determination Act. _____

_____

_____

20. Describe the Uniform Determination of Death Act. _____

_____

21. Describe the Uniform Anatomical Gift Act. _____

_____

D. Compliance Reporting

1. When a provider diagnoses a reportable disease, the state's _____ must be notified.

2. For each of the following, describe how a provider complies with the public health statutes when a communicable disease is diagnosed.

    a. If the disease is an urgent public health concern, what must be done? _____

    _____

    b. If the disease is a less urgent communicable disease, what must be done? _____

    _____

    c. How are HIV and AIDS reported by the provider? _____

    _____

    d. How might the medical assistant assist the provider with reporting communicable diseases?

    _____

3. Describe how a provider complies with the public health statutes related to wounds of violence.

   _____

   _____

4. Typically, statutes related to wounds of violence require what types of wounds to be reported?

   _____

5. Describe how a provider complies with the public health statutes related to abuse, neglect, and exploitation of children.

   _____

   _____

6. Describe how a provider complies with the public health statutes related to abuse, neglect, and exploitation of the elderly and dependent adults.

   _____

   _____

7. How does a provider handle domestic abuse situations? _____

   _____

   _____

   _____

8. When a patient is having unusual side effects from a vaccine, the provider or patient/family can file a report to the _____.

9. The _____ created the National Vaccine Injury Compensation Program that provides compensation for children injured by childhood vaccines.

10. A(n) _____ or corporate compliance is a program within a business that detects and prevents violations of state and federal laws.

11. Describe what is meant by *conflict of interest*. _____

    _____

12. Describe the process of compliance reporting related to conflicts of interest. _____

    _____

13. The _____ prohibits intentionally receiving or giving anything of value to get referrals or generate federal healthcare program business.

14. The _____ prohibits a person from submitting false or fraudulent Medicare or Medicaid claims for payment.

15. The _____ prohibits a healthcare provider from referring a Medicare patient for services to a facility in which the provider or the provider's immediate family has a financial relationship.

16. The _____ prohibits intentionally defrauding any healthcare benefit program.

17. Describe how the medical assistant should address workplace violations. _____

_____

_____

18. The _____ prohibits employment discrimination based on color, race, gender, religion, or national origin.

19. The Genetic Information Nondiscrimination Act of 2008 prohibits employment discrimination based on the _____.

20. Describe four interview topics that can put a facility at risk for discrimination lawsuits. _____

_____

_____

_____

21. List three legal interview questions. _____

_____

_____

_____

22. List three illegal interview questions. _____

_____

_____

_____

23. Describe the Americans with Disabilities Act Amendments Act (ADAAA). _____

_____

_____

24. Describe the process in compliance reporting for unsafe activities._____

_____

_____

25. Name four reasons to complete an incident report. _____

_____

_____

26. What is an incident report and what are its purposes? _____

_____

_____

27. Describe the process in compliance reporting related to incident reports. (When completing an incident report, describe three points a medical assistant should remember.)

_____

_____

_____

28. Define *risk management*. _____

_____

29. The wrong medication was given to the patient. Describe the process in compliance reporting with errors in patient care.

_____

_____

_____

CERTIFICATION PREPARATION

Circle the correct answer.

1. Which state law provides legal protection for those assisting an injured person during an emergency?
   a. Uniform Anatomical Gift Act
   b. Good Samaritan Act
   c. Patient Self-Determination Act
   d. GINA

2. Which act makes organ donation easier?
   a. Uniform Determination of Death Act
   b. National Organ Transplant Act
   c. Uniform Anatomical Gift Act
   d. Patient Self-Determination Act

3. Which act requires most healthcare institutions to inform patients of their rights to make decisions and the facility's policies about advance directives?
   a. Uniform Determination of Death Act
   b. National Organ Transplant Act
   c. Uniform Anatomical Gift Act
   d. Patient Self-Determination Act

4. Which HIPAA standard requires healthcare facilities, insurance companies, and others need to protect patient information that is electronically stored and transmitted?
   a. Standard 1 related to transactions and code sets
   b. Standard 2 related to the Privacy Rule
   c. Standard 3 related to the Security Rule
   d. Standard 4 related to unique identifiers

5. Which means individually identifiable health information stored or transmitted by covered entities or business associates?
   a. Permission
   b. PHI
   c. Covered entities
   d. Limited data set

6. Under HIPAA, healthcare providers, health (insurance) plans, and claims clearinghouses must transmit PHI electronically. What are they called?
   a. Covered entities
   b. PHI
   c. Business associates
   d. Permission

7. Under HIPAA, which is a reason for releasing or disclosing patient information?
   a. De-identify
   b. Business associates
   c. PHI
   d. Permission

8. Which psychotherapy notes are held at a higher level of confidentiality?
   a. Prescriptions for medications treating mental health disorders
   b. Results of the clinical tests related to mental health disorders
   c. Types and frequency of treatments ordered for mental health disorders
   d. What the patient said during the session and the provider's analysis of the statements and the situation

9. Which question is illegal during an interview?
   a. "Are you eligible to work in this state?"
   b. "Can you perform the essential job functions of a medical assistant with or without reasonable accommodation?"
   c. "When did you move to the United States?"
   d. "Can you work on weekends?"

10. Which act expanded the meaning and interpretation of the definition of disability and included people with cancer, diabetes, attention-deficit/hyperactivity disorder, learning disabilities, and epilepsy?
    a. ADA
    b. OSHA
    c. ADAAA
    d. Stark Law

WORKPLACE APPLICATIONS

1. The billing department supervisor at Walden-Martin Family Medical Clinic wants to hire ACE Coders to assist with the billing processes. Answer the following questions using this scenario.

   a. Who is the covered entity? _____

   b. Who is the business associate?_____

   c. What must be in done before the business associate obtains patient information? _____

   _____

   d. Can the business associates have unlimited access to all patient information? Explain why or why not.

   _____

   _____

2. Mrs. Smith asked Bella to call and talk with her daughter, Rosie. Mrs. Smith wanted Bella to tell Rosie the results of her blood test. Mrs. Smith stated that Rosie was a nurse and would understand the information. Can Bella give Mrs. Smith's information to Rosie? If not, what could be done so Rosie could get the information?

   _____

   _____

3. Mr. Green had before-and-after pictures taken as he was going through bariatric surgery and weight loss. He requests that these pictures be given to his new provider. What is the typical process to transfer pictures to another agency?

   _____

   _____

4. Mr. Thomas is a 39-year-old dependent adult. During the rooming process, the medical assistant suspects that Mr. Thomas is a victim of neglect. What should the medical assistant do?

_____

_____

INTERNET ACTIVITIES

1. Using the internet, research your state's disease reporting public health statutes. Create a poster presentation, PowerPoint presentation, or paper summarizing the reporting process for each category of diseases (e.g., urgent public health concern, less urgent, and HIV and AIDS). List three diseases for the urgent and less urgent categories.

2. Using the internet, review the Child Welfare Information Gateway website (www.childwelfare.gov) for content related to your state. You can also use government websites from your state. Create a poster presentation, PowerPoint presentation, or paper summarizing child protection in your state. Focus on related statutes, the reporting process, and who mandatory reporters are.

3. Using the internet, research prevention of elder abuse, neglect, and exploitation. Focus on resources in your state. Briefly summarize your findings and cite the websites used.

Procedure 4.1 Protecting a Patient's Privacy

Name _____ Date _____ Score _____

Tasks: Apply HIPAA rules, and protect a patient's privacy. Demonstrate sensitivity to a patient and his rights.

Scenario: Ken Thomas (date of birth [DOB] 10/25/61) saw Jean Burke N.P. (nurse practitioner) this past week. He was diagnosed with acute leukemia after several tests. You work with N.P. Burke and were involved with arranging Ken's tests. Today, Ken's adult child, Alex Thomas, calls you. Alex wants to know what is going on with Ken. You look at Ken's health record and see that Alex is not on the disclosure authorization form or a medical records release form. Per the facility's policy, for information to be given to a patient's family, a disclosure authorization form must be completed.

   Later, Ken calls and asks why you didn't update Alex on his condition. He sounds upset while he is talking with you.

Equipment and Supplies:
* Patient record
* Disclosure authorization form (electronic or paper) (See Figure 4.2)

Standard: Complete the procedure and all critical steps in _____ minutes with a minimum score of 85% within two attempts (*or as indicated by the instructor*).

Scoring: Divide the points earned by the total possible points. Failure to perform a critical step, indicated by an asterisk (*), results in grade no higher than an 84% (*or as indicated by the instructor*).

Time: Began_____ Ended_____ Total minutes: _____

Steps:	Point Value	Attempt 1	Attempt 2
1. Using the scenario, role-play the situation with a peer. You are the medical assistant and just realized that Alex is not on the release form. 　a. Be professional and respectful as you apply HIPAA to the situation. *(Refer to the Checklist for Affective Behaviors - Respect.)*	15*		
2. Inform Alex that his name is not on a disclosure authorization form. Discuss the purpose of the disclosure authorization form.	15		
3. Explain to Alex how you would be able to give him information. Encourage Alex to talk with his father about the situation.	10*		
4. (Your peer should now be Ken.) When Ken calls, be professional and respectful as you hear his complaints. Keep your voice even and do not raise the volume.	10		
5. Inform Ken that you understand his frustration. Explain why you could not give information to Alex. 　a. Show sensitivity to his feelings and his rights. *(Refer to the Checklist for Affective Behaviors - Sensitivity.)*	15*		
6. Discuss with Ken how you could prepare the disclosure authorization form. Make plans for how Ken would sign the form.	15		
7. Document the phone call with Alex and Ken. Describe the facts and the plan to complete the release form.	20*		
Total Points	**100**		

Checklist for Affective Behaviors

Affective Behavior	Directions: Check behaviors observed during the role-play.				
Respect	**Negative, Unprofessional Behaviors**	**Attempt** 1	2	**Positive, Professional Behaviors**	**Attempt** 1	2
	Rude, unkind			Courteous		
	Disrespectful, impolite			Polite		
	Unwelcoming			Welcoming		
	Brief, abrupt			Took time with patient		
	Unconcerned with person's dignity			Maintained person's dignity		
	Negative nonverbal behaviors			Positive nonverbal behaviors		
	Other:			Other:		
Sensitivity	Distracted; not focused on the other person			Focused full attention on the other person		
	Judgmental attitude; not accepting attitude			Nonjudgmental, accepting attitude		
	Failed to clarify what the person verbally or nonverbally communicated			Used summarizing or paraphrasing to clarify what the person verbally or nonverbally communicated		
	Failed to acknowledge what the person communicated			Acknowledged what the person communicated		
	Rude, discourteous			Pleasant and courteous		
	Disregards the person's dignity and rights			Maintains the person's dignity and rights		
	Other:			Other:		

Grading for Affective Behaviors		Point Value	Attempt 1	Attempt 2
Does not meet Expectation	• Response was disrespectful and/or insensitive. • Student demonstrated more than 2 negative, unprofessional behaviors during the interaction.	0		
Needs Improvement	• Response was disrespectful and/or insensitive. • Student demonstrated 1 or 2 negative, unprofessional behaviors during the interaction.	0		
Meets Expectation	• Response was respectful and sensitive; no negative, unprofessional behaviors observed. • More practice is needed for behavior to appear natural and for student to appear comfortable and at ease.	15		

Occasionally Exceeds Expectation	• Response was respectful and sensitive; no negative, unprofessional behaviors observed. • At times student appeared comfortable and at ease; but more practice is needed for behavior to become natural and consistent with a professional medical assistant.	15			
Always Exceeds Expectation	• Response was respectful and sensitive; no negative, unprofessional behaviors observed. • Student's behaviors appeared natural and comfortable. Behaviors are consistent with a professional medical assistant.	15			

Documentation

Comments

CAAHEP Competencies	Steps
X.P.2.a. Apply HIPAA rules in regard to: privacy	1-3, 6
X.A.1. Demonstrate sensitivity to patient rights	5
ABHES Competencies	**Steps**
4. Medical Law and Ethics b. Institute federal and state guidelines when: 1) Releasing medical records or information	Entire procedure
4.f. Comply with federal, state, and local health laws and regulations as they relate to healthcare settings	1-3, 6
4.h. Demonstrate compliance with HIPAA guidelines, the ADA Amendments Act, and the Health Information Technology for Economic and Clinical Health (HITECH) Act	1-3, 6

Procedure 4.2   Completing a Release of Record Form for a Release of Information

Name _____ **Date** _____ **Score** _____

Tasks: Apply HIPAA rules, and complete a release of record form for a release of information.

Scenario: Aaron Jackson was seen at Walden Hospital for a high fever. You need to help Aaron's mother complete a record release form so his record from the emergency department visit can be sent to the clinic. She needs to request all records from the visit on the first of this month. The clinic information is on the form. The release will expire in 1 month.

Aaron's information	**Walden Hospital's information**
DOB: 10/17/2011 **SSN:** 164-72-4618 **Address:** 555 McArthur Avenue, Anytown, AL 12345-1234 **Phone:** (123) 814-7844 **Mother:** Patricia Jackson	**Address:** Walden Hospital 123 Healing Way Anywhere, AL 12345-1234 **Phone:** (123) 814-4563 **Fax:** (123) 814-6544

Equipment and Supplies:
- Records release form (electronic or paper) (See Work Product 4.1)
- Patient record

Standard: Complete the procedure and all critical steps in _____ minutes with a minimum score of 85% within two attempts (*or as indicated by the instructor*).

Scoring: Divide the points earned by the total possible points. Failure to perform a critical step, indicated by an asterisk (*), results in grade no higher than an 84% (*or as indicated by the instructor*).

Time: Began_____ Ended_____ Total minutes: _____

Steps:	Point Value	Attempt 1	Attempt 2
1. Using the medical record release form, insert the patient information (Work Product 4.1). Add the patient's name, DOB, and social security number (SSN). Include the current address and phone number that is found in the patient record. If an electronic form is used, select the correct patient and the fields will auto-populate.	10*		
2. Complete the parts of the form that specify who authorizes the release and who is to release the information.	15*		
3. Check the box(es) of the information that needs to be released. If required, write in what other records need to be released.	15*		
4. Add the date of the visit. Add the name and contact information for the facility where the records need to be sent.	15*		
5. Indicate how the released information will be used.	15		
6. Indicate when the authorization should expire. Proofread the form for accuracy. If using an electronic form, save the form to the patient's record. Print the form so the mother can sign.	10		

7.	During a role-play with the patient's mother, explain what the provider is requesting. Ensure she can understand and read English. Have the mother read the form.	10		
8.	Ask the mother if she has any questions. Answer any questions and then explain where she needs to sign if she agrees with the documentation.	10		
	Total Points	**100**		

Comments

CAAHEP Competencies	Step(s)
X.P.2.b. Apply HIPAA rules in regard to: release of information	Entire procedure
ABHES Competencies	**Step(s)**
4. Medical Law and Ethics b. Institute federal and state guidelines when: 1) Releasing medical records or information	Entire procedure
4. f. Comply with federal, state, and local health laws and regulations as they relate to healthcare settings	Entire procedure
4.h. Demonstrate compliance with HIPAA guidelines, the ADA Amendments Act, and the Health Information Technology for Economic and Clinical Health (HITECH) Act	Entire procedure

Work Product 4.1   Records Release Form

Name _____   Date _____   Score _____

WALDEN-MARTIN
FAMILY MEDICAL CLINIC
1234 ANYSTREET | ANYTOWN, ANYSTATE 12345
PHONE 123-123-1234 | FAX 123-123-5678

Medical Records Release

Patient Name: _____   Date of Birth: _____

SSN: _____   Phone: _____

Address:

I, _____ authorize _____

to disclose/release the following information (check all applicable):

☐ All Records   ☐ Abstract/Summary

☐ Laboratory/pathology records   ☐ Pharmacy/prescription records

☐ X-ray/radiology records   ☐ Other

☐ Billing records

Note: If these records contain any information from previous providers or information about HIV/AIDS status, cancer diagnosis, drug alcohol abuse, or sexually transmitted disease, you are hereby authorizing disclosure of this information. A copy of this signed authorization must be given to the individual.

These records are for services provided on the following date(s):_____

Please send the records listed above to (use additional sheets if necessary):

Name: _____   Phone: _____

Address: Fax: _____

The information may be used/disclosed for each of the following purposes:

☐ At patient's request   ☐ For employment purposes

☐ For patient's health care   ☐ Other

☐ For payment/insurance

This authorization shall expire no later than: _____ or upon the following event _____ , and may not be valid for greater than one year from the date of signature for medical records.

I understand that after the custodian of records discloses my health information, it may no longer be protected by federal privacy laws. I understand that this authorization is voluntary and I may refuse to sign this authorization which will not affect my ability to obtain treatment; receive payment; or eligibility for benefits unless allowed by law. By signing below I represent and warrant that I have authority to sign this document and authorize the use or disclosure of protected health information and that there are no claims or orders that would prohibit, limit, or otherwise restrict my ability to authorize the use or disclosure of this protected health information.

_____

Patient signature
(or patient's personal representative)

Date

_____

Printed name of patient representative

Representative's authority to sign for patient
(i.e. parent, guardian, power of attorney, executor)

Procedure 4.3   Perform Disease Reporting

Name _____ **Date** _____ **Score** _____

Tasks: Research the state's disease reporting public health statutes and complete the disease reporting paperwork based on public health statutes. Document the activity in the patient's health record.

Scenario: Jean Burke N.P. received the test results for Ken Thomas. He tested positive for gonorrhea. She wants you to file the report with the public health department. Here is the information from his health record and the clinic. For any missing information, follow the instructor's directions or make it up if no directions were provided.

Patient Information	Provider and Lab Information	Health Record Information
Ken Thomas 398 Larkin Avenue Anytown, AL 12345-1234 Anycounty k.thomas@anytown.mail Phone: (123) 784-1118 DOB: 10/25/61 Race: Multiple races Ethnicity: Unknown Marital status: Single Living with Sandy Brown, who was not treated	Provider: Jean Burke, N.P. Walden-Martin Family Medical Clinic 1234 Anystreet Anytown, AL 12345-1234 Phone: (123) 123-1234 Fax: (123) 123-5678 Lab: Walden-Martin Family Medical Clinic Lab	Diagnosis: Gonorrhea Symptoms: Started 5 days ago, greenish discharge from penis, burning with urination Test: Urine specimen was collected yesterday; gonorrhea nucleic acid amplification test NAAT test done yesterday, results are positive Treatment: Patient treated today with ceftriaxone 250 mg intramuscular (IM) single dose and azithromycin 1 g orally single dose

Equipment and Supplies:
- Computer with internet access and printer
- Patient record (see table with information)
- Black pen

Standard: Complete the procedure and all critical steps in _____ minutes with a minimum score of 85% within two attempts (*or as indicated by the instructor*).

Scoring: Divide the points earned by the total possible points. Failure to perform a critical step, indicated by an asterisk (*), results in grade no higher than an 84% (*or as indicated by the instructor*).

Time: Began_____ Ended_____ Total minutes: _____

Steps:	Point Value	Attempt 1	Attempt 2
1. Using the internet, search for the disease reporting procedure in your state's public health department or similar facility. Read the procedure.	10		
2. Identify which form is required based on the patient's diagnosis. Print the form.	10		

3.	Use a black pen to complete the form. Neatly complete the patient's demographic information section using the information from the health record.	25		
4.	Complete the diagnosis, symptoms, testing, and treatment information.	25		
5.	Complete the rest of the form. Review the form for accuracy. Make any changes required before submitting the form to the instructor.	20		
6.	Document in the patient's health record that the disease reporting paperwork was completed and submitted	10		
Total Points		**100**		

Documentation

Comments

CAAHEP Competencies	Step(s)
X.P.5. Perform compliance reporting based on public health statutes	Entire procedure
ABHES Competencies	**Step(s)**
4. Medical Law and Ethics f. Comply with federal, state, and local health laws and regulations as they relate to healthcare settings	Entire procedure
4.b.2) Entering orders in and utilizing electronic health records	6

Procedure 4.4   Report Illegal Activity

Name _____   Date _____   Score _____

Task: Report an illegal activity in the healthcare setting following proper protocol.

Scenario: Today, you witnessed a coworker, Sally Brown, taking medical samples from the supply cabinet. You see her sticking them in her purse. She sees you and states, "This was the same medication I had to pay $200 for the last time I was sick. I don't see why we need to pay for medications when we have samples that we give free to patients. We should be able to use them too." You know the facility's professional policy prohibits taking medical samples from the sample cabinet for personal reasons.

Facility's Compliance Reporting Protocol:
Walden-Martin Family Medical Clinic's Compliance Program has a phone number and email address for employees to report suspected violations, suspected illegal activity, fraud, abuse, theft, and workplace safety concerns. Concerns can be left on the voicemail or emailed without fear of retribution or retaliation. Please include as many details as possible, including date(s), names, and the situation.

    Any employee who seeks retribution or retaliation against another employee for reporting an offense needs to be aware of criminal penalties for such actions.

Equipment and Supplies:
- Computer with email and internet access or phone
- Instructor's email address or voicemail phone number
- Pen and paper
- Facility's compliance reporting protocol (See box)

Standard: Complete the procedure and all critical steps with a minimum score of 85% within two attempts (*or as indicated by the instructor*).

Scoring: Divide the points earned by the total possible points. Failure to perform a critical step, indicated by an asterisk (*), results in grade no higher than an 84% (*or as indicated by the instructor*).

Steps:	Point Value	Attempt 1	Attempt 2
1. Read the facility's corporate compliance reporting protocol.	10		
2. Using the paper and pen, write down the facts of what you witnessed.	10		
3. Using the paper and pen, compose the message you want to email or leave on the voicemail for the compliance office.	30		
4. Proofread the message and make any changes required. Make sure to include the date, names of people involved, and the details of the situation.	20		
5. Using your email or phone, send a message to the corporate compliance office. Use the email address or phone number provided by your instructor.	30		
Total Points	100		

Comments

CAAHEP Competencies	Step(s)
X.P.6. Report an illegal activity in the healthcare setting following proper protocol	Entire procedure
ABHES Competencies	**Step(s)**
4. Medical Law and Ethics f. Comply with federal, state, and local health laws and regulations as they relate to healthcare settings	Entire procedure

Procedure 4.5   Complete Incident Report

Name _____ Date _____ Score _____

Task: Complete an incident report form for a medication error.

Scenario: Johnny Parker (DOB 06/15/10) saw Jean Burke N.P. for a well-child visit. Johnny is off schedule with his hepatitis B vaccine series and today he is to get his last hepatitis B booster. You (a medical assistant) prepare the medication and give the injection in his right deltoid muscle. Later in the day, you realize that hepatitis B was out of stock for 1 week. You must have given a hepatitis A booster to Johnny. You realized that you failed to read the label three times during the preparation of the medication. You reported the mistake to Jean Burke N.P. and your supervisor. Your supervisor called Lisa Parker, Johnny's mother. They will come back next week for the hepatitis B vaccine. You need to complete the incident report.

Equipment and Supplies:
- Incident Report form (Work Product 4.2) and black pen or computer with an internet and SimChart for the Medical Office (SCMO)

Standard: Complete the procedure and all critical steps in _____ minutes with a minimum score of 85% within two attempts (*or as indicated by the instructor*).

Scoring: Divide the points earned by the total possible points. Failure to perform a critical step, indicated by an asterisk (*), results in grade no higher than an 84% (*or as indicated by the instructor*).

Time: Began_____ Ended_____ Total minutes: _____

Steps:	Point Value	Attempt 1	Attempt 2
1. SCMO method: Access SCMO and enter the Simulation Playground. If a popup window appears, select "Return to previous session with saved patient information" and click Start. On the Calendar screen, click on the Form Repository icon. Click on Office Forms on the left Info Panel and select Incident Report. For both methods: Accurately complete the information from the date down to the reason for the patient's visit.	20		
2. For both methods: Specify the incident description, immediate action and outcome, and contributing factors, and fill in the prevention boxes. Provide as much detail as possible. Be honest and concise with your facts.	20		
3. For both methods: Complete the reported by, position, and contact phone number sections. Your information should be in these fields. Make up a contact phone number.	20		
4. For both methods: Complete the other persons involved, position, and contact phone number sections. Jean Burke's information should be in these fields. Make up her contact phone number.	20		
5. For both methods: Review the form for accuracy. Make any changes required before submitting the form to the instructor. (For the SCMO method: Save or print the form based on your instructor's directions.)	20		
Total Points	**100**		

Comments

CAAHEP Competencies	Step(s)
X.P.7. Complete an incident report related to an error in patient care	Entire procedure
ABHES Competencies	**Step(s)**
4. Medical Law and Ethics e. Perform risk management procedures	Entire procedure

Work Product 4.2   Incident Report Form

Name _____   Date _____   Score _____

WALDEN-MARTIN
FAMILY MEDICAL CLINIC
1234 ANYSTREET | ANYTOWN, ANYSTATE 12345
PHONE 123-123-1234 | FAX 123-123-5678

Incident Report

Date: _____   Time: _____

Incident Type: ☐ Staff   ☐ Patient   ☐ Visitor   ☐ Equipment/Property

Witness: ☐ Staff   ☐ Patient   ☐ Visitor

Department: _____   Exact Location: _____

Medical Team: _____

Patient Reason for Visit: _____   Medication Incident: ☐ Yes ☐ No

Incident Description:

Immediate Actions and Outcome:

Contributing Factors:

Prevention:

Next of kin / guardian notified / patient?   ☐ Yes   ☐ No   ☐ N/A   Medical staff notified?   ☐ Yes   ☐ No   ☐ N/A

Reported By: _____   Position: _____

Contact Phone Number: _____

Other Persons Involved: _____   Position: _____

Contact Phone Number: _____

Medical Report (Document patient's assessment and list investigations and treatments):

_____

Provider: _____   Designation: _____

Provider Signature: _____   Date/Time: _____

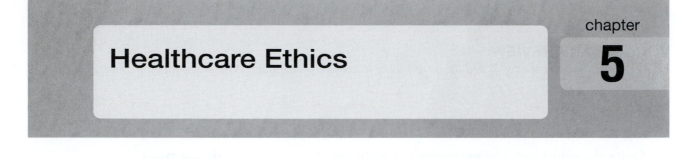

Healthcare Ethics

chapter

5

CAAHEP Competencies	Assessment
V.C.17.c. Discuss the theories of: Kübler-Ross	Skills and Concepts – C. 18 a-e; Certification Preparation – 6
X.C.7.e. Define: Uniform Anatomical Gift Act	Skills and Concepts – C. 26
X.C.7.f. Define: living will/advanced directives	Vocabulary Review – D. 3, 5; Certification Preparation – 7
X.C.7.g. Define: medical durable power of attorney	Vocabulary Review – D. 4
X.C.7.h. Define: Patient Self Determination Act (PSDA)	Skills and Concepts – C. 20
XI.C.1.a. Define: ethics	Vocabulary Review – D. 1; Certification Preparation – 1
XI.C.1.b. Define: morals	Vocabulary Review – D. 2; Certification Preparation – 2
XI.C.2. Differentiate between personal and professional ethics	Skills and Concepts – A. 3; Certification Preparation – 3
XI.C.3. Identify the effect of personal morals on professional performance	Skills and Concepts – A. 2
XI.P.1. Develop a plan for separation of personal and professional ethics	Procedure 5.1
XI.P.2. Demonstrate appropriate response(s) to ethical issues	Procedure 5.2
XI.A.1. Recognize the impact personal ethics and morals have on the delivery of healthcare	Procedure 5.1, 5.2
ABHES Competencies	Assessment
4. Medical Law and Ethics g. Display compliance with the Code of Ethics of the profession	Skills and Concepts – A. 6 Procedure 5.1, 5.2

VOCABULARY REVIEW

Using the word pool on the right, find the correct word to match the definition. Write the word on the line after the definition.

Group A

1. Codes of conduct stated by an employer or professional association _____

2. Basic units of heredity _____

3. Rod-shaped structures found in the cell's nucleus; they contain genetic information _____

4. A set of rules about good and bad behavior _____

5. An individual's code of conduct _____

6. The freedom to determine one's own actions and decisions _____

7. People who study the ethical effect of biomedical advances _____

8. To treat patients fairly and give them care that is due and appropriate _____

9. To do good _____

10. To do no harm _____

Word Pool
- autonomy
- chromosomes
- beneficence
- code of ethics
- justice
- genes
- nonmaleficence
- professional ethics
- personal ethics
- bioethicists

Group B

1. The inability to get pregnant after 1 year of unprotected intercourse _____

2. Nonreproductive cells; they do not include sperm and egg cells _____

3. Cells can make copies of themselves _____

4. Sperm and egg cells _____

5. Cells can develop into specialized cells _____

6. The process of creating a genetically identical biological entity _____

7. The entire genetic makeup of an organism _____

8. A branch of medicine involved with using patients' genomic information as part of their clinical care _____

9. A branch of pharmacology that studies the genetic factors that influences a person's response to a medication _____

10. The manipulation of genetic material in cells to change hereditary traits or produce a specific result _____

Word Pool
- genomic medicine
- differentiate
- self-renew
- genome
- cloning
- genetic engineering
- somatic cells
- germline cells
- pharmacogenomics
- infertility

Group C

1. A competent adult can appoint a person to make healthcare decisions in the event he or she is unable to do so

   _____

2. Withholding a life-saving treatment (e.g., feeding tube) and letting the person die _____

3. A branch of knowledge, learning, or instruction; for instance, medicine, nursing, social work, and physical therapy

   _____

4. Incorporating the most current and valid research results into the practice of healthcare, thus providing the best patient care

   _____

5. Latin for "father of the country" _____

6. Involves removing egg cells from a female's ovaries, fertilizing them with sperm outside of the body, and then implanting the fertilized egg in the uterus _____

7. To help relieve the symptoms of a serious illness

   _____

8. A type of palliative care for people who have about 6 months or less to live _____

9. Bringing to an end _____

10. The act of killing a person who is suffering from an incurable disease _____

11. To preserve by freezing at low temperatures

    _____

12. A physician who has graduated from medical school and is finishing specialized clinical training _____

13. An immature ovum _____

14. A person who acts on behalf of another person or takes the place of another person _____

15. A group composed of members from a variety of disciplines that analyzes ethical issues _____

16. Any procedure where nonhuman cells, tissues, or organs are implanted or infused into a person _____

Word Pool
- cessation
- evidence-based practices
- in-vitro fertilization
- *parens patriae*
- healthcare proxy
- discipline
- xenotransplantation
- resident
- hospice
- euthanasia
- cryopreservation
- oocyte
- ethics committees
- passive euthanasia
- palliative
- surrogate

Group D

Define each word or phrase.

1. Ethics: _____

   _____

2. Morals: _____

   _____

3. Advance directives: _____

    _____

4. Medical durable power of attorney:_____

    _____

5. Living will:_____

    _____

ABBREVIATIONS

Write out what each of the following abbreviations stands for.

1. AMA _____

2. CEJA _____

3. AAMA _____

4. GMOs _____

5. FDA _____

6. ART _____

7. IUI _____

8. STI _____

9. NHI _____

10. PSDA _____

11. DNR _____

12. CPR _____

13. POLST _____

14. UDDA _____

15. UAGA _____

16. NOTA _____

17. OPTN _____

SKILLS AND CONCEPTS

Answer the following questions. Write your answer on the line or in the space provided.

A. Personal and Professional Ethics

1. Describe morals and their impact on a person's life._____

_____

_____

2. Identify the effect of personal morals on professional performance. _____

_____

_____

3. Describe the difference between personal and professional ethics. _____

_____

_____

4. What are codes of ethics and who publishes them? _____

_____

_____

5. What is the CEJA and what does it do?_____

_____

_____

6. Summarize the Medical Assisting Code of Ethics. _____

_____

_____

7. How can a medical assistant approach a situation if it involves his or her biases? _____

_____

_____

8. When looking for employment, why is it important to consider one's biases before applying for certain jobs?

_____

_____

B. Principles of Healthcare Ethics

1. List the four ethical principles. _____

    _____

2. How can a medical assistant follow the ethical principle of autonomy when caring for patients?

    _____

    _____

3. How can a medical assistant follow the ethical principle of nonmaleficence when caring for patients?

    _____

    _____

4. How can a medical assistant follow the ethical principle of beneficence when caring for patients?

    _____

    _____

5. How can a medical assistant follow the ethical principle of justice when caring for patients?

    _____

    _____

C. Ethical Issues

1. Describe the positions of advocates and opponents of human cloning. _____

    _____

    _____

2. What is the Human Genome Project and what resulted from the project? _____

    _____

    _____

3. _____ can identify issues with a person's chromosomes, genes, or proteins.

4. List seven types of genetic testing. _____

    _____

    _____

5. When using pharmacogenomics, what is an advantage to a patient? _____

    _____

6. What are the two main categories of stem cells? _____

    _____

7. What is gene therapy? _____

_____

8. _____ technique can remove, add, or alter sections of the gene.

9. Describe the difference between genome editing of somatic cells and germline cells. _____

_____

_____

10. What is an ethical issue that may arise with assistive reproductive technology?_____

_____

_____

11. Describe CEJA's opinion on assistive reproductive technology._____

_____

_____

12. Discuss the CEJA's opinion on gamete donation. _____

_____

_____

13. What power does the *parens patriae* doctrine gives the courts? _____

_____

_____

14. Discuss the CEJA's opinion on parental refusal of treatment._____

_____

_____

15. Describe the difference between open and closed adoptions. _____

_____

_____

16. What are the Safe Haven Infant Protection laws and what is the main goal of these laws? _____

_____

_____

17. Describe CEJA's opinion on confidential healthcare for minors. _____

_____

_____

18. Describe the following stages of grief and dying of Elisabeth Kübler-Ross' theory.

    a. Denial: _____

    _____

    b. Anger: _____

    _____

    c. Bargaining: _____

    _____

    d. Depression: _____

    _____

    e. Acceptance: _____

    _____

19. Where can hospice care be provided? _____

    _____

20. Describe the importance of the Patient Self-Determination Act (PSDA). _____

    _____

21. What does the CEJA encourage providers to do regarding advance directives? _____

    _____

22. Besides addressing different types of advance directions, list five other topics found on advance directive forms.

    _____

    _____

    _____

23. Describe importance of the Uniform Determination of Death Act. _____

    _____

    _____

24. What is CEJA's opinion on physician-assisted suicide and euthanasia? _____

    _____

    _____

25. What should a person do if he or she wants to be a potential organ donor at death? _____

    _____

    _____

26. Describe the Uniform Anatomical Gift Act. _____

_____

_____

27. The _____ established the Organ Procurement and Transplant Network (OPTN).

CERTIFICATION PREPARATION

Circle the correct answer.

1. Which term means "rules of conduct that differentiate between acceptable and unacceptable behavior"?
   a. Ethics
   b. Justice
   c. Morals
   d. Code of ethics

2. Which term means "internal principles that distinguish between right and wrong"?
   a. Ethics
   b. Morals
   c. Justice
   d. Nonmaleficence

3. _____ are codes of conduct stated by an employer or professional association.
   a. Personal ethics
   b. Morals
   c. Professional ethics
   d. Code of ethics

4. Which means "to do no harm"?
   a. Autonomy
   b. Justice
   c. Nonmaleficence
   d. Beneficence

5. What is the process of creating a genetically identical biological entity?
   a. Genetic engineering
   b. Cloning
   c. Genetic testing
   d. Pharmacogenetics

6. Which Kübler-Ross stage of grief and dying involves the person refusing to accept the fact?
   a. Anger
   b. Depression
   c. Bargaining
   d. Denial

7. Which advance directive provides instructions about life-sustaining medical treatment to be administered or withheld when the patient has a terminal condition?
   a. Medical durable power of attorney
   b. Healthcare proxy
   c. Living will
   d. Organ donation

8. Which advance directive allows a competent adult to appoint a person (called a *proxy* or *agent*) to make healthcare decisions in the event he or she is unable to do so?
   a. Medical durable power of attorney
   b. Healthcare proxy
   c. Living will
   d. Organ donation

9. Which is the type of euthanasia where the patient consents to the action?
   a. Active
   b. Passive
   c. Voluntary
   d. Involuntary

10. Which act established a national registry for organ matching and also made it a criminal act to exchange organs for transplant for something of value?
    a. Patient Self-Determination Act
    b. Uniform Anatomical Gift Act
    c. Uniform Determination of Death Act
    d. National Organ Transplant Act

WORKPLACE APPLICATIONS

1. Mrs. Johnson called Walden-Martin Family Medical Clinic and Daniela answered the phone. Mrs. Johnson requested an appointment. She stated that she has experienced sleep changes, difficulty concentrating, sadness, and appetite changes since her husband died. Based on what you have read in this chapter, what might be occurring with Mrs. Johnson?

_____

_____

2. Jean is graduating from a medical assistant program. During her practicum, she heard about the dangers of narcotic medications. She does not believe that patients should receive narcotic medications. Jean is an advocate of alternative medications and feels there are reasonable alternatives to narcotic medications. How should Jean approach finding a job, given her bias?

_____

_____

3. Jan, a certified medical assistant, was discussing advance directives with a patient. The patient asked Jan to explain the importance of advance directives. How would you explain the importance of advance directives?

_____

_____

_____

INTERNET ACTIVITIES

1. Using the internet, research your state's advance directive forms. Create a poster presentation, PowerPoint presentation, or paper summarizing the topic areas on the advance directive forms. Cite your resource(s).

2. Using the internet, research your state's Safe Haven laws for children. If your state does not have these laws, select a state that does. Create a poster presentation, PowerPoint presentation, or paper summarizing the Safe Haven laws. Focus on related statutes, maximum age of the child, and locations where the child can be brought. Cite your resource(s).

3. Using the internet, research an ethical issue. Create a poster presentation, PowerPoint presentation, or paper summarizing your findings. In your project, summarize the ethical issue and provide the advocates' and opponents' views of the issue.

Procedure 5.1 Developing an Ethics Separation Plan

Name _____ Date _____ Score _____

Task: To develop a plan for separation of personal and professional ethics.

Scenario: You are working at WMFM Clinic. Your provider sees many children, including teens. New state laws allow for confidential healthcare for minors. The agency has now adopted policies and procedures to allow providers to see teens 16 years or older without parental consent. The teens can be seen for sexually transmitted infections (STIs) and reproductive issues (including birth control). All health records related to these visits are confidential, meaning parents cannot be told about their child's visit.

Your personal belief is that parents should always be allowed to know what is occurring with their children. They are responsible for the child until age 18 and they pay the bills. You also believe that children (younger than 18) are too young to be in an intimate relationship. This type of activity should only be for adults in a committed relationship. You don't believe in birth control.

Equipment and Supplies:
- Paper and pen
- Medical Assisting Code of Ethics (see box in the textbook)

Standard: Complete the procedure and all critical steps with a minimum score of 85% within two attempts (*or as indicated by the instructor*).

Scoring: Divide the points earned by the total possible points. Failure to perform a critical step, indicated by an asterisk (*), results in grade no higher than an 84% (*or as indicated by the instructor*).

Steps/Criteria:	Point Value	Attempt 1	Attempt 2
1. Read the Medical Assisting Code of Ethics. Write down key themes or phrases.	15		
2. Using the scenario, write down the professional ethics involved in the situation.	15		
3. Using the scenario, write down the personal ethics involved in the situation.	15		
4. Compare the lists. Identify the personal ethics that conflict with the Code of Ethics and the professional ethics of the agency.	15		
5. For each area of conflict, create a plan on how you will separate your personal and professional ethics. Remember as a professional, you need to follow the professional ethics of the agency and the profession. Address how will you handle the situation and what your options would be if you were in the situation.	20*		
6. Describe how the personal ethics and morals in this scenario would impact patient care and the delivery of healthcare. • Describe how a medical assistant's personal ethics and morals could impact how that person provides care. • Describe how patient care may be altered or not up to the standard of care required. • Describe how a medical assistant could respond in a professional manner and maintain the standard of care and personal integrity.	20*		
Total Points	**100**		

Comments

CAAHEP Competencies	Steps
XI.P.1. Develop a plan for separation of personal and professional ethics	5
XI.A.1. Recognize the impact personal ethics and morals have on the delivery of healthcare	6
ABHES Competencies	**Steps**
4. Medical Law and Ethics g. Display compliance with the Code of Ethics of the profession	5

Procedure 5.2 Demonstrate Appropriate Response to Ethical Issues

Name _____ Date _____ Score _____

Tasks: Identify ethical issues and demonstrate appropriate and professional responses. Recognize the impact personal ethics and morals have on the delivery of healthcare.

Scenario 1: You are working at WMFM Clinic. You are responsible for collecting payments from patients. Mr. Smythe, who is visually impaired, paid for his visit in cash. He gives you $500 for a $402 bill. You make change and give him a receipt. At the end of the day, you notice that you have $60 more than what you should have and some of the bills were mixed up in the cashbox. You realize you gave Mr. Smythe the incorrect amount of money.

Scenario 2: You are setting up a laceration repair tray for Dr. Martin to use. As you are preparing the sterile equipment, one of the instruments gets contaminated. You know Dr. Martin urgently needs the tray. You realize the contamination can cause an infection.

Equipment and Supplies:
- Paper and pen

Standard: Complete the procedure and all critical steps in _____ minutes with a minimum score of 85% within two attempts (*or as indicated by the instructor*).

Scoring: Divide the points earned by the total possible points. Failure to perform a critical step, indicated by an asterisk (*), results in grade no higher than an 84% (*or as indicated by the instructor*).

Time: Began_____ Ended_____ Total minutes: _____

Steps:	Point Value	Attempt 1	Attempt 2
1. Read both scenarios. Identify and write down the ethical issues involved.	20		
2. With a peer, role-play Scenario 1. Your peer should be the supervisor in this scenario. Demonstrate a professional and appropriate ethical response to this situation. a. Explain the situation to the supervisor. b. Describe how you felt the error occurred and who received the incorrect change. c. Explain how you would like to handle the situation and correct the error.	30		
3. With a peer, role-play Scenario 2. Your peer should be the provider in this scenario. During the role-play, demonstrate a professional and appropriate ethical response to this situation.	30		
4. In a written response, discuss the potential implications for the patient's health related to not reporting or correcting the error.	20		
Total Points	**100**		

- Ethical issue(s) identified in Scenario 1:

- Ethical issue(s) identified in Scenario 2:

- Discuss the potential implication to the patient's health related to not reporting or correcting the error.

Comments

CAAHEP Competencies	Step(s)
XI.P.2. Demonstrate appropriate response(s) to ethical issues	1-3
XI.A.1. Recognize the impact personal ethics and morals have on the delivery of healthcare	4
ABHES Competencies	**Step(s)**
4. Medical Law and Ethics g. Display compliance with the Code of Ethics of the profession	Entire procedure

Introduction to Anatomy and Medical Terminology

CAAHEP Competencies

V.C.9. Identify medical terms labeling the word parts	Skills and Concepts – A. 7, 8, 10
I.C.1. Describe structural organization of the human body	Skills and Concepts – B. 1-20
I.C.2. Identify body systems	Skills and Concepts – B. 11-21
I.C.3.a. Describe: body planes	Skills and Concepts – G. 1
I.C.3.b. Describe: directional terms	Skills and Concepts – D. 1-10
I.C.3.c. Describe: quadrants	Skills and Concepts – F. 1-7
I.C.3.d. Describe: body cavities	Skills and Concepts – E. 1-6
V.C.10. Define medical terms and abbreviations related to all body system	Vocabulary Review – A. 1-11, B. 1-12; Abbreviations – 1-46
I.C.7. Describe the normal function of each body system	Skills and Concepts – B. 10-21
I.C.4. List major organs in each body system	Skills and Concepts – B. 10-21, E. 1-6, F. 1-7
I.C.4. List major organs in each body system	Skills and Concepts – B. 10-21, E. 1-6, F. 1-7

ABHES Competencies

3. Medical Terminology

a. Define and use the entire basic structure of medical terminology and be able to accurately identify the correct context (i.e., root, prefix, suffix, combinations, spelling and definitions)	Skills and Concepts – A. 7, 8, 10
b. Build and dissect medical terminology from roots and suffixes to understand the word element combinations	Skills and Concepts – A. 10
c. Apply medical terminology for each specialty	Vocabulary Review – A. 1-11, B. 1-12; Skills and Concepts – C. 2-15, D. 1-10
d. Define and use medical abbreviations when appropriate and acceptable	Abbreviations – 1-46

VOCABULARY REVIEW

Using the word pool, find the correct word to match the definition. Write the word on the line after the definition.

Group A

1. A rapidly dividing cancer cell that has little to no similarity to normal cells _____

2. Protein substances produced in the blood or tissues in response to a specific antigen that destroy or weaken the antigen; part of the immune system _____

3. A broad dome-shaped muscle used for breathing that separates the thoracic and abdominopelvic cavities

   _____

4. Word parts that appear at the beginning of terms

   _____

5. Process of viewing living tissue that has been removed for the purpose of diagnosis or treatment _____

6. The "subjects" of most terms; they consist of the word root with its respective combining vowel _____

7. Substances that stimulate the production of an antibody when introduced into the body; include toxins, bacteria, viruses, and other foreign substances _____

8. Rod-shaped structures found in the cell's nucleus; they contain genetic information _____

9. Words used in healthcare whose definitions must be memorized without the benefit of word parts _____

10. Describes how malignant tissue looks like the normal tissue it came from; poorly _____ means it does not look like the normal tissue, and well _____ means it looks like the normal tissue

    _____

11. Word parts that appear at the end of terms

    _____

Word Pool
- prefixes
- antigens
- biopsy
- differentiated
- anaplastic
- diaphragm
- combining forms
- suffixes
- antibodies
- nondecodable terms
- chromosomes

Group B

1. A specially trained doctor who diagnoses and treats cancer _____

2. A cell division process by which two daughter cells are formed from one parent cell; each daughter has a complete copy of parent's chromosomes _____

3. Located between cells _____

4. Wavelike motion _____

5. A disease-causing organism _____

6. Structures inside of the cell that have specific functions to maintain the cell _____

7. An examination using a scope with a camera attached to a long, thin tube that can be inserted into the body _____

8. A physician specially trained in the nature and cause of disease _____

9. Contraction of the muscles causing the narrowing of the inside tube of the vessel _____

10. Substances created by microorganisms, plants, or animals and poisonous to humans _____

11. Study of disease _____

12. The internal environment of the body that is compatible with life; a steady state that is created by all the body systems working together to provide a consistent and unvarying internal environment _____

Word Pool
- endoscopy
- pathogen
- homeostasis
- vasoconstriction
- mitosis
- pathology
- toxins
- intercellular
- peristalsis
- oncologist
- organelle
- pathologist

ABBREVIATIONS
Write out what each of the following abbreviations stands for.

1. CARD _____

2. AAMA _____

3. AAMT _____

4. AMA _____

5. ER _____

6. DNA _____

7. IM _____

8. CABG _____

9. TURP _____

10. AP _____

11. PA _____

6. Define the acronym CARD.

    C _____

    A _____

    R _____

    D _____

7. Using Table 6.1 in the textbook, write the definition of the following combining forms.

    a. ot/o _____

    b. cardi/o_____

    c. nephr/o_____

    d. hepat/o _____

    e. ophthalm/o _____

    f. neur/o _____

8. Using Table 6.2 in the textbook, write the definition of the following suffixes.

    a. -logy _____

    b. -plasty _____

    c. -algia _____

    d. -itis _____

    e. -tomy _____

    f. -scope_____

9. With only a few exceptions, how many spelling rules apply to decodable medical terms?_____

    _____

    _____

10. Using Tables 6.1 through 6.10 in your textbook, decode and define the following terms. Label the word
    parts as prefix, combining form, or suffix.

    a. ophthalmology_____

    _____

    b. otoplasty _____

    _____

    c. gastralgia_____

    _____

    d. cardiomegaly _____

                 _____

    e. osteomalacia _____

                 _____

    f. cephalic _____

                 _____

    g. gastroptosis _____

                 _____

    h. spirometer _____

                 _____

    i. splenectomy _____

                 _____

    j. pericardium _____

                 _____

11. For each of the following words, write the plural form using the rules discussed in your textbook under the heading Singular/Plural Rules.

    a. esophagus _____

    b. larynx _____

    c. fornix _____

    d. pleura _____

    e. diagnosis _____

    f. myocardium _____

    g. cardiomyopathy _____

    h. hepatitis _____

ANATOMY REVIEW

B. Structural Organization of the Body

1. The _____ is the basic unit of life.

2. _____ is the process where one cell splits into two identical daughter cells.

3. At what stage of mitosis is the genetic information replicated? _____

4. List the four phases of mitosis. _____

_____

_____

5. _____ is the jelly-like substance that surrounds the organelles and fills the cell.

6. What causes the rough appearance of the rough endoplasmic reticulum? _____

_____

_____

7. _____ is a group of similar cells from the same source that together carry out a specific function.

8. List the four types of tissues and give two examples of each.

a. epithelial _____

_____

_____

b. connective _____

_____

_____

c. muscle _____

_____

_____

d. nervous _____

_____

_____

9. _____ is a structure composed of two or more types of tissue.

10. A(n) _____ is composed of several organs and their related structures.

11. Which body system contains veins, arteries, and blood? _____

12. Which body system is involved with the breakdown, digestion, and absorption of nutrients?
_____

13. Which body system includes the pituitary and the thyroid glands? _____

14. Receiving and processing information and controlling body structures to maintain homeostasis are roles of which body system? _____

15. Which body system is involved with heat production, support, protection, and movement?
_____

16. Which body system provides immunity and maintains fluid balance? _____

17. Protection and temperature regulation are some roles of the _____ system; hair and nails are also structures in this system.

18. Which body system is involved with producing children and hormones? _____

19. Delivering oxygen to cells and ridding the body of carbon dioxide are two major roles of which body system? _____

20. Which body system is involved with gathering information from vision, hearing, balance, smell, and taste? _____

21. Eliminating nitrogenous waste from the body and maintaining fluid and electrolytes are important roles for which body system? _____

22. Put the following in order from the simplest to the most complex: organism, organs, cells, body systems, tissue

_____

C. Surface Anatomy Terminology

1. Describe the anatomical position._____

_____

_____

2. *Cervical* refers to the:_____

3. *Frontal* pertains to the: _____

4. *Ocular* refers to the:_____

5. *Axillary* refers to the:_____

6. *Coxal* pertains to the:_____

7. *Sternal* pertains to the: _____

8. *Antecubital* pertains to the:_____

9. *Carpal* refers to the: _____

10. *Femoral* pertains to the:_____

11. *Patellar* pertains to the: _____

12. *Pedal* pertains to the:_____

13. *Acromial* refers to the: _____

14. *Lumbar* pertains to the: _____

15. *Plantar* pertains to the: _____

D. Positional and Directional Terminology

1. *Deep* or *internal* refers to: _____

2. *Anterior* or *ventral* pertains to the:_____

3. *Inferior* or *caudad* pertains to: _____

4. Opposite of *anterior* and refers to the back:_____

5. Pertains to the midline: _____

6. *Contralateral* refers to the:_____

7. *Distal* refers to:_____

8. Pertains to carrying toward a structure: _____

9. Pertains to near the origin: _____

10. Using the directional and positional terms listed in this chapter, write four sentences that use a term in reference to the body. Use four different terms. Example: The fingers are distal to the elbows.

    _____

    _____

    _____

    _____

E. Body Cavities

1. Name the two cavities that make up the dorsal body cavity. _____

    _____

2. Name the two cavities that make up the ventral body cavity._____

    _____

3. Describe the cranial cavity. _____

    _____

    _____

4. Describe the spinal cavity._____

    _____

    _____

5. Describe the thoracic cavity. _____

    _____

    _____

6. Discuss the two cavities that make up the abdominopelvic cavity. _____

_____

_____

F. Abdominopelvic Quadrants and Regions

1. Describe the imaginary lines for the abdominopelvic quadrants. _____

_____

2. List three organs found in the right upper quadrant. _____

_____

3. List three organs found in the left upper quadrant. _____

_____

4. List three organs found in the left lower quadrant. _____

_____

5. List three organs found in the right lower quadrant. _____

_____

6. Describe the advantage of using the abdominal regions compared to the abdominopelvic quadrants.

_____

_____

7. Using the grid below, create a table showing the locations of the nine abdominal regions. In each box, indicate the region and one organ found in that region.

Right hypochondriac region	Epigastric region	Left hypochondriac region
Right lumbar region	Umbilical region	Left lumbar region
Right iliac region	Hypogastric region	Left iliac region

G. Body Planes

1. Using your own words, describe the following planes.

   a. Midsagittal or median plane _____

   _____

   b. Coronal or frontal plane _____

   _____

   c. Transverse or horizontal plane _____

   _____

H. Acid-Base Balance

1. What is the pH of an acidic solution? _____

2. What is the pH of a basic or alkaline solution? _____

3. For the body to maintain homeostasis, what pH range must be maintained in the blood? _____

   _____

4. What three things must work together to maintain the acid-base range in the body? _____

   _____

I. Pathology Basics

1. Describe the difference between the following terms.

   a. Prevalence and incidence _____

   _____

   b. Morbidity and mortality_____

   _____

   c. Acute and chronic _____

   _____

   d. Signs and symptoms _____

   _____

2. List five predisposing factors for disease._____

   _____

3. Describe the difference between noncommunicable diseases and communicable diseases. _____

   _____

4. Describe the characteristics of a benign tumor. _____

_____

5. Describe the characteristics of a malignant tumor. _____

_____

_____

6. Describe grade and stage. _____

_____

_____

CERTIFICATION PREPARATION

Circle the correct answer.

1. What does *–ptosis* mean?
   a. Abnormal condition of softening
   b. Abnormal condition of hardening
   c. Prolapse, drooping, sagging
   d. Enlargement

2. What is the prefix that means between?
   a. inter-
   b. intra-
   c. peri-
   d. pre-

3. What is the prefix that means above, upon?
   a. endo-
   b. hypo-
   c. sub-
   d. epi-

4. What two prefixes mean within?
   a. endo-, intra-
   b. epi-, inter-
   c. ante-, per-
   d. peri-, trans-

5. What is the structural organization of the body from the simplest to the most complex?
   a. Organism, body system, tissues, organs, and cells
   b. Cells, organs, tissues, and body systems
   c. Cells, tissues, organs, body systems, and organism
   d. Cells, tissues, body systems, organs, and organism

6. Which body system produces hormones that circulate in the blood to target tissues that stimulate a particular action?
   a. Cardiovascular
   b. Endocrine
   c. Blood
   d. Integumentary

7. Which body system includes joints, tendons, ligaments, and cartilage?
   a. Integumentary
   b. Nervous
   c. Reproductive
   d. Musculoskeletal

8. Which plane divides the body into the front and back portions?
   a. Frontal plane
   b. Median plane
   c. Midsagittal plane
   d. Transverse plane

9. _____ pertains to the middle and _____ pertains to the side.
   a. Anterior; posterior
   b. Superior; inferior
   c. Ipsilateral; contralateral
   d. Medial; lateral

10. Which cavity is part of the ventral body cavity and contains the heart and lungs?
    a. Spinal cavity
    b. Thoracic cavity
    c. Abdominopelvic cavity
    d. Cranial cavity

WORKPLACE APPLICATIONS

1. Harry is a new student who thinks he might want to become a physician's assistant. He likes to practice decoding terms. What does the combining form mean in each of the following terms?

   a. Cystocele means herniation of the _____ .

   b. Ophthalmology is the study of the _____ .

   c. Otalgia is pain in the _____ .

   d. Osteoma is a tumor in a(n) _____ .

   e. Hepatitis is inflammation of the _____ .

2. Daniela was discussing directional terms with a peer in her class. She was explaining the importance of using directional terms in healthcare. Describe why directional terms are useful when documenting healthcare information.

   _____

   _____

   _____

3. Describe the organizational structure of the body. _____

   _____

   _____

   _____

   _____

INTERNET ACTIVITIES

1. Select one of the causes of disease (e.g., genetics, infectious pathogen). Using online resources, find four diseases that are initiated by that specific cause of disease. Research each disease and the cause of the disease. Create a paper, poster presentation, PowerPoint presentation, or infographic based on your research.

2. Using online resources, research grading and staging of cancers. Create a short paper or PowerPoint describing the difference between grading and staging.

3. Research the difference between acid and base. Write a half-page summary on the importance of the acid-base balance of the body.

4. Research and create a list of the most prevalent forms of cancer for males and females in the United States.

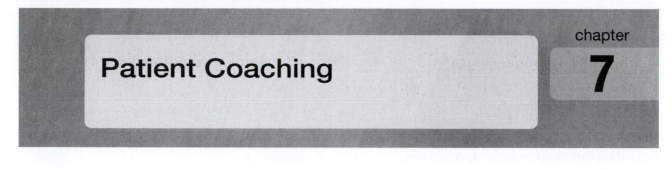

Patient Coaching

CAAHEP Competencies	Assessment
V.C.6.a. Define coaching a patient as it relates to: health maintenance	Skills and Concepts – A. 4-5; Certification Preparation – 2
V.C.6.b. Define coaching a patient as it relates to: disease prevention	Skills and Concepts – A. 2-3
V.C.6.c. Define coaching a patient as it relates to: compliance with treatment plan	Skills and Concepts – A. 6-7
V.C.6.d. Define coaching a patient as it relates to: community resources	Skills and Concepts – A. 9
V.C.6.e. Define coaching a patient as it relates to: adaptations relevant to individual patient needs	Skills and Concepts – A. 8; C. 16
V.C.12. Define patient navigator	Skills and Concepts – H. 3
V.C.13. Describe the role of the medical assistant as a patient navigator	Skills and Concepts – H. 4-5
V.C.17.b. Discuss the theories of: Erikson	Skills and Concepts – C. 17a-h; Workplace Applications – 1a-h; Certification Preparation – 6
V.C.17.c. Discuss the theories of: Kübler-Ross	Skills and Concepts – B. 1a-e, 2, 3a-e; Certification Preparation – 4
V.P.9. Develop a current list of community resources related to patients' healthcare needs	Procedure 7.2
V.P.10. Facilitate referrals to community resources in the role of a patient navigator	Procedure 7.2
V.P.4.c. Coach patients regarding: disease prevention	Procedure 7.1
V.P.5.b. Coach patients appropriately considering: developmental life stage	Procedure 7.1
V.P.5.c. Coach patients appropriately considering: communication barriers	Procedure 7.1
X.P.3. Document patient care accurately in the medical record	Procedure 7.1, 7.2

ABHES Competencies	Assessment
5. Human Relations b. 3) List organizations and support groups that can assist patients and family members of patients experiencing terminal illnesses	Procedure 7.2
5.d. Adapt care to address the developmental stages of life	Procedure 7.1
8.h. Teach self-examination, disease management and health promotion	Procedure 7.1
8.i. Identify community resources and Complementary and Alternative Medicine practices (CAM)	Procedure 7.2
8.j. Make adaptations for patients with special needs (psychological or physical limitations)	Procedure 7.1
8.k. Make adaptations to care for patients across their lifespan	Procedure 7.1

VOCABULARY REVIEW

Using the word pool on the right, find the correct word to match the definition. Write the word on the line after the definition.

1. The act of sticking to something _____
2. The process of gaining new knowledge or skills through instruction, experience, or study _____
3. Patients are taking the right dose at the right times as prescribed by the provider _____
4. "Doing" domain _____
5. Bringing to an end _____
6. Involves mental processes of recall, application, and evaluation _____
7. Provides personalized patient- and family-centered care in a team-based environment _____
8. "Feeling" domain _____
9. The act of following through on a request or demand _____
10. The inability to feel or experience pleasure during a pleasurable activity _____
11. A person who identifies patients' barriers, works closely with the healthcare team and patients, and guides the patients through the healthcare system _____
12. The set of behaviors, ideas, and customs shared by a specific group of people, which distinguishes the members from other people _____
13. Focuses on the interrelationship among the physical, mental, social, and spiritual aspects of the person's life _____

Word Pool
- medication adherence
- compliance
- cessation
- culture
- adherence
- care coordination
- holistic
- learning
- patient navigator
- affective domain
- anhedonia
- cognitive domain
- psychomotor domain

ABBREVIATIONS

Write out what each of the following abbreviations stands for.

1. Td _____

2. HZV _____

3. PCV13 _____

4. Tdap _____

5. PPSV23 _____

6. BSE _____

7. TSE _____

8. UV _____

9. PSA _____

10. DRE _____

11. AAA _____

12. PHQ-9 _____

13. NIH _____

14. CDC _____

15. ADA _____

16. AHA _____

17. HPV _____

18. DEA _____

19. FDA _____

20. gFOBT _____

21. FIT _____

22. MT-sDNA _____

SKILLS AND CONCEPTS

Answer the following questions. Write your answer on the line or in the space provided.

A. Coaching

1. Describe coaching in your own words. _____

_____

_____

2. Define coaching a patient as it relates to disease prevention. _____

_____

3. List two types of disease prevention coaching a medical assistant may provide. _____

_____

4. Define coaching a patient as it relates to health maintenance. _____

_____

5. List two types of health maintenance coaching a medical assistant may provide. _____

_____

6. Define coaching a patient as it relates to compliance with a treatment plan. _____

_____

_____

7. How can coaching help increase a patient's compliance or adherence to the treatment plan? _____

_____

_____

8. Define coaching a patient as it relates to adaptations (special needs) relevant to individual patient needs.

_____

_____

_____

9. Define coaching a patient as it relates to community resources. _____

_____

_____

_____

B. Making Changes for Health

1. Describe the following grief and dying stages by Kübler-Ross.

   a. Denial _____

   _____

   b. Anger _____

   _____

   c. Bargaining _____

   _____

  d. Depression _____

   _____

  e. Acceptance _____

   _____

2. Describe how grieving may impact a patient's compliance with a treatment plan._____

  _____

  _____

3. List adaptive interactions used for each stage of grief and dying.

  a. Denial _____

   _____

  b. Anger_____

   _____

  c. Bargaining_____

   _____

  d. Depression _____

   _____

  e. Acceptance _____

   _____

4. What does the health belief model help to explain? _____

  _____

5. Briefly describe the three parts of the health belief model. _____

  _____

  _____

  _____

  _____

C. Basics of Teaching and Learning

1. Briefly describe the cognitive domain of learning. _____

  _____

  _____

  _____

2. Related to the cognitive domain, list four ways a medical assistant can help patients remember critical information.

   _____

   _____

   _____

3. List three cognitive teaching strategies._____

   _____

4. List two barriers to the cognitive learning domain. _____

   _____

5. List three strategies a medical assistant could use to adapt to the cognitive learning barriers._____

   _____

   _____

6. Briefly describe the psychomotor domain of learning._____

   _____

7. Related to the psychomotor domain, list four ways a medical assistant can help patients remember critical information.

   _____

   _____

   _____

8. List two psychomotor teaching strategies. _____

   _____

9. List two barriers to the psychomotor learning domain. _____

   _____

10. List a strategy a medical assistant could use to adapt to the psychomotor learning barriers. _____

    _____

11. Briefly describe the affective domain of learning. _____

    _____

12. Related to the affective domain, list two ways a medical assistant can help patients remember critical information.

    _____

    _____

13. List two affective teaching strategies. _____

_____

14. List three barriers to the affective learning domain. _____

_____

15. List a strategy a medical assistant could use to adapt to the affective learning barriers. _____

_____

16. List two things a medical assistant should consider when adapting coaching to a patient._____

_____

_____

17. Describe the goals of each of Erikson's psychosocial development stages.

   a. Trust versus mistrust _____

_____

   b. Autonomy versus shame and doubt_____

_____

   c. Initiative versus guilt _____

_____

   d. Industry versus inferiority _____

_____

   e. Identity versus role confusion _____

_____

   f. Intimacy versus isolation _____

_____

   g. Generativity versus stagnation _____

_____

   h. Ego integrity versus despair _____

_____

18. Describe three strategies to use when communicating with patients who have impaired vision.

_____

_____

_____

_____

19. Describe five strategies to use when communicating with patients who have impaired hearing.

    _____

    _____

20. Describe three strategies to use when communicating with patients who have language barriers.

    _____

    _____

21. How should a medical assistant start the coaching process?_____

    _____

    _____

D. Coaching on Disease Prevention

1. List three common disease prevention coaching topics a medical assistant may provide._____

    _____

    _____

2. Describe cough etiquette._____

    _____

    _____

E. Coaching on Health Maintenance and Wellness

1. What is the purpose of self-exams? _____

    _____

    _____

2. Women with an average risk of breast cancer should start having yearly mammograms between age
    _____ and _____.

3. About half of men diagnosed with testicular cancer are between _____ and _____ years of age.

4. _____ is the most dangerous type of skin cancer.

5. List three risk factors for skin cancer. _____

    _____

    _____

6. List four symptoms of oral cancer._____

    _____

    _____

7. People age 18-39 years should have a blood pressure check every _____ to _____ years.

8. Adults with no history of high cholesterol should have it checked every _____ years.

9. Adults 45 years old and older with normal risk should have a stool screening test every _____ or _____ years depending on the test and a colonoscopy every _____ years.

10. A dental exam and cleaning are recommended _____.

11. For women ages 30-65, a Pap test is recommended every 5 years if the _____ test is also done.

12. Type 2 diabetes mellitus screening should be done every _____ years starting at age 18.

13. List three risk factors for hepatitis C. _____

_____

_____

14. An alcoholic drink is classified as a(n) _____ of beer, a(n) _____ of wine, or a(n) _____ of liquor.

15. List five common signs of drug abuse. _____

_____

_____

16. Intimate partner violence includes what behaviors? _____

_____

_____

17. Describe common signs of elder abuse and neglect for each of the following categories.

   a. Physical abuse _____

   _____

   b. Emotional abuse _____

   _____

   c. Neglect _____

   _____

F. Coaching on Diagnostic Tests

1. List two advantages of the Cologuard Stool DNA test over the guaiac fecal occult blood test. _____

_____

_____

_____

2. A patient needs to undergo a CT scan that requires contrast medium.

   a. What questions should the medical assistant ask the patient? _____

   _____

   _____

   b. List common patient instructions. _____

   _____

   _____

3. A patient needs to undergo a magnetic resonance imaging (MRI).

   a. What questions should the medical assistant ask the patient? _____

   _____

   _____

   b. List common patient instructions. _____

   _____

   _____

4. A patient needs to undergo mammography.

   a. What questions should the medical assistant ask the patient? _____

   _____

   _____

   b. List common patient instructions. _____

   _____

   _____

5. A patient needs to have a Pap test. List common patient preparation instructions. _____

   _____

   _____

G. Coaching on Treatment Plans

1. What type of information do patients need to know when taking medications at home? _____

   _____

   _____

   _____

   _____

H. Care Coordination

1. Describe the goals of care coordination in the ambulatory care setting. _____

_____

_____

2. Name four advantages of care coordination. _____

_____

_____

3. Define *patient navigator*. _____

_____

_____

_____

4. Describe the role of the medical assistant as a patient navigator. _____

_____

_____

5. For care coordination/patient navigation, with what areas could the medical assistant assist the patient?

_____

_____

_____

6. Describe types of community resources. _____

_____

_____

_____

CERTIFICATION PREPARATION

Circle the correct answer.

1. Coaching provides patients with
   a. skills.
   b. knowledge.
   c. support and confidence.
   d. all of the above.

2. Providing patients with information on routine screenings and showing patients how to do self-exams is what type of coaching?
   a. Disease prevention
   b. Health maintenance
   c. Diagnostic tests
   d. Specific needs

3. Providing patients with information on hygiene practices, recommended vaccines, and nicotine cessation is what type of coaching?
    a. Disease prevention
    b. Health maintenance
    c. Diagnostic tests
    d. Specific needs

4. When a patient is experiencing sadness and uncertainty when grieving, what stage of Kübler-Ross' theory is the person in?
    a. Denial
    b. Anger
    c. Bargaining
    d. Depression

5. Language barriers are barriers to learning in the _____ domain.
    a. psychomotor
    b. affective
    c. cognitive
    d. a and c

6. According to Erikson's theory, an adolescent is in which stage?
    a. Identity versus role confusion
    b. Intimacy versus isolation
    c. Industry versus inferiority
    d. Generativity versus stagnation

7. What colorectal cancer screening test requires no patient preparation and consists of a computer analysis that checks the stool for cancer and precancerous cells?
    a. gFOBT
    b. FIT
    c. PET
    d. MD-sDNA

8. Which imaging procedure uses x-rays to create pictures of cross-sections of the patient's body?
    a. X-ray
    b. Computed tomography scan
    c. Magnetic resonance imaging
    d. Mammography

9. What diagnostic test provides an x-ray picture of the breasts and is used to find tumors?
    a. X-ray
    b. Computed tomography scan
    c. Magnetic resonance imaging
    d. Mammography

10. What diagnostic test uses high-frequency sound waves to create an image of the organs and structures?
    a. Ultrasound
    b. Computed tomography scan
    c. Magnetic resonance imaging
    d. Mammography

WORKPLACE APPLICATIONS

1. Working in family medicine, Suzanne works with people of all ages. Describe tips to remember when coaching/working with patients of the following ages.

    a. 1-year-old _____

    _____

    b. 2-year-old _____

    _____

    c. 5-year-old _____

    _____

    d. 8-year-old _____

    _____

    e. 14-year-old _____

    _____

f. 30-year-old _____

_____

g. 72-year-old _____

_____

_____

2. Suzanne is coaching a patient about the early warning signs of malignant melanoma. Describe the ABCDE rule.

_____

_____

_____

_____

INTERNET ACTIVITIES

1. Using the FDA website (www.fda.gov), research "disposal of unused medications" in the home environment. Create a poster, PowerPoint, or paper summarizing your research. Focus on these areas:
    a. Using authorized collectors for disposal (e.g., take-back programs)
    b. Disposal in household trash
    c. Disposing of fentanyl patches

2. Using the CDC website (www.cdc.gov), research recommended immunizations for children. Create a poster, PowerPoint, or paper summarizing your research. Focus on five recommended childhood immunizations and address the following for each:
    a. Name of immunization
    b. Why is it recommended or what does it prevent?
    c. Schedule of the vaccine (or the ages when a child should receive the immunization)
    d. Side effects of the vaccine

3. Using the CDC website (www.cdc.gov), research recommended immunizations. Create a poster, PowerPoint, or paper summarizing your research. Focus on immunizations prior to, during, and after pregnancy.
    a. What is recommended? Why is it recommended?
    b. What is not recommended?

Procedure 7.1 Coach a Patient on Disease Prevention

Name _____ Date _____ Score _____

Tasks: Coach a patient on the recommended vaccinations for his or her age. Adapt coaching for the patient's communication barriers and developmental life stage. Document the coaching in the patient's health record.

Scenario: You are working with Dr. David Kahn. You need to room Charles Johnson (date of birth [DOB]: 03/03/1958) and his record indicates he has not been seen in several years. Charles has a significant hearing loss and he communicates by signing. His wife interprets for him. You look in his health record and see that he is due for influenza, Td, and recombinant zoster (shingles) vaccines. Per the provider's request (order), you need to coach adult patients on potential vaccines they are due for during the initial rooming process.

Directions: Role-play this scenario with two other peers.

Equipment and Supplies:
- VIS (available at http://www.immunize.org/vis/)
- Patient's health record

Standard: Complete the procedure and all critical steps in _____ minutes with a minimum score of 85% within two attempts (*or as indicated by the instructor*).

Scoring: Divide the points earned by the total possible points. Failure to perform a critical step, indicated by an asterisk (*), results in grade no higher than an 84% (*or as indicated by the instructor*).

Time: Began _____ Ended _____ Total minutes: _____

Steps:	Point Value	Attempt 1	Attempt 2
1. Wash hands or use hand sanitizer.	5		
2. Greet the patient. Identify yourself. Verify the patient's identity with full name and date of birth. Explain what you will be doing.	10		
3. Arrange the chairs so the patient can see both you and the person signing. Speak slowly. Pause as needed to allow person signing to finish with the last statement. Look at the patient when communicating.	15		
4. Use simpler language when talking. Speak clearly. Communicate with dignity and respect. Allow time for the patient to respond. Listen to the patient's concerns.	15*		
5. Ask the patient if he has received vaccines somewhere else over the past few years.	5		
Scenario update: Patient has not seen any healthcare providers over the last few years. The only vaccines received were given in this facility. 6. Describe the vaccines that are due. Use the VIS for each vaccine as you coach the patient on the purpose of the vaccine.	15*		
Scenario update: The patient knows the shingles vaccine is not covered and costs more than $200. He refuses the shingles vaccines and he does not believe in getting the influenza vaccine. He is interested in getting the Td vaccine. 7. Ask the patient which vaccines he is interested in getting. If he refuses, be respectful of his choice. Any reason he gives for the refusal should be communicated to the provider.	15*		

8.	Document the coaching in the patient's health record. Include the provider's name, what was taught, how the patient responded, and any vaccines refused.	20		
	Total Points	100		

Documentation

Comments

CAAHEP Competencies	**Step(s)**
V.P.4.c. Coach patients regarding: disease prevention	6, 7
V.P.5.b. Coach patients appropriately considering: developmental life stage	4
V.P.5.c. Coach patients appropriately considering: communication barriers	3, 4
X.P.3. Document patient care accurately in the medical record	8
ABHES Competencies	**Step(s)**
5.d. Adapt care to address the developmental stages of life	4
8.h. Teach self-examination, disease management and health promotion	6
8.j. Make adaptations for patients with special needs (psychological or physical limitations)	3, 4
8.k. Make adaptations to care for patients across their lifespan	4

Procedure 7.2   Develop a List of Community Resources and Facilitate Referrals

Name _____ Date _____ Score _____

Tasks: As a patient navigator, develop a current list of community resources that meet the patient's health-care needs. Discuss the resources with the patient and facilitate referrals to the chosen resources.

Scenario 1: Robert Caudill (DOB: 10/31/1940) was just diagnosed with dementia. He currently lives with his daughter, Ruby, who works full-time. Ruby is feeling overwhelmed with being his only caregiver and realizes that she needs to find someone to care for her father while she is working.

Scenario 2: Leslie Green (DOB 08/03/03) just tested positive for pregnancy. She does not feel that she has a support system to help her make decisions.

Scenario 3: Ella Rainwater's husband of 30 years died suddenly 1 month ago. Ella (DOB: 07/11/1959) stated that she feels alone and has no one to talk to. Her daughter feels that she needs the support of others who have gone through the same thing.

Directions: Role-play these scenarios with another peer. The peer will be the family member or patient during the first part of the role-play and then the community resource agency representative during the second part.

Equipment and Supplies:
- Computer with internet or a telephone book
- Paper and pen
- Community Resource Referral Form (Work Product 7.1) or referral form
- Patient's health record

Standard: Complete the procedure and all critical steps in _____ minutes with a minimum score of 85% within two attempts (*or as indicated by the instructor*).

Scoring: Divide the points earned by the total possible points. Failure to perform a critical step, indicated by an asterisk (*), results in grade no higher than an 84% (*or as indicated by the instructor*).

Time: Began_____ Ended_____ Total minutes: _____

Steps:	Point Value	Attempt 1	Attempt 2
1. Using the scenario, identify the possible types of community resources that would assist each patient or family. Identify three different types of resources (e.g., medical equipment, support group) that would meet each patient's needs.	5		
2. Using the internet or the phone book, identify two local resources for each of the three kinds of resources (i.e., find two assisted living resources, two medical equipment suppliers, etc.). Make a list of six resources for the patient and family. Include the following: a. Organization's name b. Address and contact information c. Summary of the services provided d. Cost and other relevant information	30		

3.	*Role-play the scenario indicated by the instructor*: Provide the patient or family member with the list of six resources. Describe the services offered and any costs.	15*		
4.	Allow the patient or family member time to review the services. Answer any questions.	10		
5.	Use professional, tactful verbal and nonverbal communication as you work with the patient or family member.	10*		
6.	*Role-play making the community referral(s)*: Have the patient or family member decide on two or more services they are interested in. Complete the referral document (Work Product 7.1). Have the patient provide any additional information required on the form. Call the community resource agency and provide the referral information to the representative (a peer).	20*		
7.	Document the patient education and the referrals in the health record.	10		
	Total Points	100		

Documentation

Comments

CAAHEP Competencies	Step(s)
V.P.9. Develop a current list of community resources related to patients' healthcare needs	1, 2
V.P.10. Facilitate referrals to community resources in the role of a patient navigator	3-6
X.P.3. Document patient care accurately in the medical record	7
ABHES Competencies	**Step(s)**
5. Human Relations b.3) List organizations and support groups that can assist patients and family members of patients experiencing terminal illnesses	1, 2
8.i. Identify community resources and Complementary and Alternative Medicine practices (CAM)	1, 2

Work Product 7.1   Community Resource Referral Form

To be used with Procedure 7.2.

Name _____   Date _____   Score _____

Patient's Name:	Date of Birth:

Community Resource Information:

Agency: _____   Contact Name: _____
Address: _____   Phone number: _____
_____   Website: _____

Services
Provided:

Agency: _____   Contact Name: _____
Address: _____   Phone number: _____
_____   Website: _____

Services
Provided:

Agency: _____   Contact Name: _____
Address: _____   Phone number: _____
_____   Website: _____

Services
Provided:

Agency: _____   Contact Name: _____
Address: _____   Phone number: _____
_____   Website: _____

Services
Provided:

chapter

8

Technology

CAAHEP Competencies	Assessment
VI.C.8. Differentiate between electronic medical records (EMR) and a practice management system	Skills and Concepts – D. 3 a-b; Certification Preparation – 4-5
VI.C.11. Explain the importance of data back-up	Skills and Concepts – E. 5-6
XII.C.7.b. Identify principles of: ergonomics	Skills and Concepts – C. 2 a-f, 3

ABHES Competencies	Assessment
7. Administrative Procedure h. Perform basic computer skills	Procedure 8.2
8. Clinical Procedures a. Practice standard precautions and perform disinfection/sterilization techniques	Procedure 8.1

Group C

1. An itemized statement of services and costs from a healthcare facility submitted to the health (insurance) plan for payment

   _____

2. Money collected for providing a product or service

   _____

3. An interconnection between systems _____

4. An electronic record of health-related information about an individual that can be created, gathered, managed, and accessed by authorized clinicians and staff members within a single healthcare organization; also called _EMR_

   _____

5. A collection of data or program records stored as a unit with a specific name _____

6. Unauthorized user who attempts to break into computer networks

   _____

7. Malicious software designed to damage or disrupt a system

   _____

8. The electronic exchange of information between two agencies to accomplish financial or administrative healthcare activities

   _____

9. Individually identifiable health information stored or transmitted by covered entities or business associates

   _____

10. Identification of potential threats of computer network breaches, for which action plans for corrective actions are instituted

    _____

Word Pool
- security risk analysis
- malware
- interface
- hacker
- claim
- file
- revenue
- electronic medical record
- protected health information
- electronic transactions

Group D

1. The computer process of changing encrypted text to readable or plain text after a user enters a secret key or password

   _____

2. A person or business that provides a service to a covered entity that involves access to PHI _____

3. Each employee with network access must log in using a unique password _____

4. Devices attached to the monitor that allow visualization of the screen contents only if the user is directly in front of the screen

   _____

5. Program or hardware that acts as a barrier between the network and the internet _____

6. Something designed to be used at or near where the patient is seen; point-of-care tools and apps are resources for the provider to use when working directly with the patient

   _____

7. A wireless mobile workstation _____

8. The use of electronic software to communicate with pharmacies and send prescribing information _____

9. A healthcare facility, healthcare provider, pharmacy, health (insurance) plan, or claims clearinghouse that transmits protected health information electronically _____

10. The interval of time during which something, such as hardware or software, is not functioning _____

11. Refers to remote clinical and nonclinical services, such as provider training, meetings, and continuing education

    _____

Word Pool

- point-of-care
- telehealth
- computer on wheels
- e-prescribing
- business associate
- firewall
- downtime
- covered entity
- privacy filters
- authentication
- decryption

ABBREVIATIONS

Write out what each of the following abbreviations stands for.

1. EHR _____

2. PC _____

3. OCR _____

4. GB _____

5. ISP _____

6. DSL _____

7. IT _____

8. EMR _____

9. HIPAA _____

10. ePHI _____

11. CPU _____

12. ROM _____

13. RAM _____

14. MB _____

15. HITECH _____

16. COW _____

17. CPOE _____

18. RPM _____

19. mHealth _____

20. HHR _____

SKILLS AND CONCEPTS

Answer the following questions. Write your answer on the line or in the space provided.

A. Computers in Ambulatory Care

1. List the three types of personal computers. _____

   _____

2. The PC and peripheral devices are _____.

3. List five input devices. _____

   _____

4. Describe the difference among the function, control, and special-purpose keys on keyboards.

   _____

   _____

   _____

   _____

5. List three ways to move the pointer (cursor) on the screen. _____

   _____

6. What hardware and software are used for telemedicine? _____

   _____

   _____

7. What is a patient portal? _____

   _____

8. Scanners convert images to digital text using a process called _____.

9. List four types of scanners. _____

_____

10. List three output devices. _____

_____

11. Images are created on monitors using _____; the _____ the number, the sharper the image.

12. Describe the advantages of inkjet and laser printers. _____

_____

_____

13. The _____ is the "brains" of the computer and it sits on the

_____.

14. Describe the three types of primary memory. _____

_____

_____

_____

15. When saving data to the computer, the data are saved on the _____ drive.

16. Describe cloud storage. _____

_____

_____

17. A(n) _____ is usually considered a character, such as a number, letter, or symbol.

18. Put these data storage capacities in order from smallest to largest: MB, GB, TB, KB_____

_____

19. What two things are required for a healthcare facility's computer network to access the internet?

_____

B. Maintaining Computer Hardware

1. Describe three ways to prevent computer problems. _____

_____

_____

_____

2. Describe the Security Rule's physical safeguards and list four safeguards. _____

_____

_____

3. Describe three physical safeguards that are part of workstation security. _____

_____

_____

4. Describe the Security Rule's technical safeguards and list seven safeguards. _____

_____

_____

5. Describe the data backup process. _____

_____

_____

6. What is the importance of frequently backing up the network data? _____

_____

_____

F. Continual Technology Advances in Healthcare

1. Explain e-prescribing. _____

_____

2. What is computerized provider/physician order entry (CPOE) and who is allowed to use CPOE?

_____

_____

CERTIFICATION PREPARATION

Circle the correct answer.

1. What is one kilobyte equivalent to?
   a. 1024 bytes
   b. 1024 MB
   c. 1024 GB
   d. 1024 TB

2. Which software protects computers against viruses?
   a. Database software
   b. Presentation software
   c. Anti-malware software
   d. Spreadsheet software

3. What is a physical safeguard that is used over monitors to prevent others from seeing the information?
   a. Firewalls
   b. Screen savers
   c. Authentication
   d. Privacy filters

4. Which is a type of software that allows the user to enter demographic information, schedule appointments, maintain lists of insurance payers, perform billing tasks, and generate reports?
   a. Electronic health record (EHR)
   b. Electronic medical records (EMR)
   c. Practice management
   d. Microsoft Word and Excel

5. What is an electronic version of a patient's paper record?
   a. Electronic health record (EHR)
   b. Electronic medical records (EMR)
   c. Practice management
   d. A and B

6. What are records of computer activity used to monitor users' actions within software, including additions, deletions, and viewing of electronic records?
   a. Automatic log-off
   b. Authentication
   c. Firewalls
   d. Audit trails

7. What is a program or hardware device that acts as a barrier or filter between the network and the internet?
   a. Firewalls
   b. Screen savers
   c. Authentication
   d. Privacy filters

8. What means potential threats to the computer system security are identified, the likelihood of such occurrence is determined, and additional safeguards are implemented?
   a. Firewalls
   b. Security risk analysis
   c. Authentication
   d. Privacy filters

9. What makes a strong password?
   a. Use a person's name
   b. Use eight or more characters
   c. Use a random combination of upper- and lowercase letters, numbers, and symbols
   d. B and C

10. Which is the computer memory used for loading and running programs?
    a. ROM
    b. RAM
    c. Cache
    d. Hard drive

WORKPLACE APPLICATIONS

1. As part of her role, Christiana is learning about security measures to keep the network secure and confidential. Identify the security measures described.

   a. After a period of inactivity, the workstation logs off. _____

   b. Used to encode or change the information into nonreadable or encrypted data. _____

   c. Multiple incorrect log-in attempts are flagged, and many times the account is locked. Prevents hackers from cracking passwords.

   d. Each employee is assigned a unique name or number for identifying and tracking user identity.

2. Christiana is evaluating the scanners in the reception area and the health information management department, which handles scanning documents into the electronic health records. Discuss types of scanners that might be used in both of these areas.

    _____

    _____

    _____

3. Christiana would like to have a computer with internet access available for patients to use in the reception area. What are things that she will need to consider?

    _____

    _____

INTERNET ACTIVITIES

1. Review the content of one of the patient education websites listed in the chapter. Create a poster presentation, a PowerPoint presentation, or write a paper summarizing your research.

2. Select a disease. Find two reputable patient education websites that provide information on the disease, diagnostic tests, and treatments. One of your websites must be different than those listed in the chapter. Create a poster presentation, a PowerPoint presentation, or write a paper summarizing your research and include the websites used.

3. You need to purchase a printer for your department. Research a business-size laser printer and an inkjet printer. Create a poster presentation, a PowerPoint presentation, or write a paper summarizing your research and include the websites used. Include the following points for each printer:
    a. Name and model number of the printer
    b. Cost of the printer
    c. Cost of a new printer cartridge
    d. Speed of the printer
    e. Additional features of the printer that would be useful in a business setting

Procedure 8.1 Prepare a Workstation

Name _____ Date _____ Score _____

Tasks: Perform infection control procedures and create an ergonomically friendly workstation.

Equipment and Supplies:
- Nonabrasive disinfectant (hospital grade) wipes or specially made wipes for computer hardware or as indicated by the keyboard manufacturer
- Gloves (if required for using wipes)
- User guide for keyboard or facility's infection control procedure for computer hardware
- Desktop computer with adjustable monitor
- Office chair with an adjustable seat, armrest, and backrest
- Footrest (if needed)
- Foam wrist rest
- Document holder (optional)
- Hand sanitizer (optional)

Standard: Complete the procedure and all critical steps in _____ minutes with a minimum score of 85% within two attempts (*or as indicated by the instructor*).

Scoring: Divide the points earned by the total possible points. Failure to perform a critical step, indicated by an asterisk (*), results in grade no higher than an 84% (*or as indicated by the instructor*).

Time: Began_____ Ended_____ Total minutes: _____

Steps:	Point Value	Attempt 1	Attempt 2
1. While sitting in the chair, adjust the backrest so it supports the upper body and the lumbar support area fits to the small of the back. Adjust the seat pan height so the feet are flat on the floor or footrest. Adjust the armrest to support the forearms with the shoulders in a relaxed position.	20		
2. Adjust the monitor so it is directly in front of the person and the top of the monitor is at or just below the eye level. If using a document holder, position it so it is at the same distance and height as the monitor.	20		
3. Place the keyboard at a height and an angle to allow the wrists to be in a neutral position. Position the mouse so it is at elbow level for typing. Support the wrists with a foam wrist rest.	20		
4. While sitting with your torso and neck vertically and in line, identify if everything is positioned correctly and comfortably. Make any adjustments as needed.	10		
5. Using the keyboard user guide or the facilities infection control procedure for computer hardware, determine the product to use to disinfect the keyboard. Don gloves if needed. Using a disinfectant wipe, clean the surface using friction for 5 seconds in each area. Discard gloves if worn.	20*		
6. Wash hands or use hand sanitizer before using the keyboard.	10*		
Total Points	100		

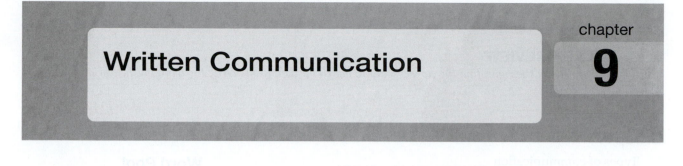

Written Communication

chapter

9

CAAHEP Competencies	Assessment
V.C.7. Recognize elements of fundamental writing skills	Vocabulary Review – A. 2-6; Skills and Concepts – A. 1-10 Certification Preparation – 1-3
V.C.8. Discuss applications of electronic technology in professional communication	Skills and Concepts – B. 1, 19
V.P.8. Compose professional correspondence utilizing electronic technology	Procedure 9.1, 9.2, 9.3, 9.4, 9.5

ABHES Competencies	Assessment
7. Administrative Procedures g. Display professionalism through written and verbal communications	Procedure 9.1, 9.2, 9.3, 9.4, 9.5, 9.6
h. Perform basic computer skills	Procedure 9.1, 9.2, 9.3, 9.4, 9.5

VOCABULARY REVIEW

Using the word pool on the right, find the correct word to match the definition. Write the word on the line after the definition.

Group A

1. Types of communication _____

2. A word or group of words that describes a noun or pronoun

   _____

3. A word or group of words that answers how, where, when, or to what extent, thus further describing a verb, adjective, or adverbs

   _____

4. Often begin with words such as *although, since, when, because,* and *if*; needs a subject and verb to be a complete sentence

   _____

5. A word that indicates a relationship or a location between a noun or pronoun and the rest of the sentence _____

6. A group of words without a subject or verb

   _____

7. Notes the initials of the person who composed the letter in uppercase followed by the initials of the person who keyed (typed) the letter in lowercase _____

8. Used to notify the letter's recipient who else received a copy of the letter _____

9. A type of software that allows the user to enter demographic information, schedule appointments, maintain lists of insurance payers, perform billing tasks, and generate reports

   _____

10. A document or file that has a preset format

    _____

Word Pool
- reference notation
- preposition
- adjective
- dependent clauses
- media
- copy notation
- practice management software
- phrase
- adverb
- template

Group B

1. A person who has written documentation that he or she can accept a shipment for another individual _____

2. An electronic record that conforms to nationally recognized standards and contains health-related information about a specific patient _____

3. The most common layout for a printed page; the height of the paper is greater than its width _____

4. Documents sent to a patient explaining that the provider is ending the physician-patient relationship and the patient needs to see another provider _____

5. The measurement around something; when referring to mail, it is the measurement around the middle of the package that is being shipped _____

6. A region or geographic area used for shipping

   _____

7. A term describing employees for whom an employer has obtained a fidelity bond from an insurance company, which will cover losses from any dishonest acts (e.g., embezzlement, theft) committed by those employees _____

Word Pool
- girth
- electronic health record
- authorized agent
- bonded
- portrait orientation
- zone
- termination letters

SKILLS AND CONCEPTS

Answer the following questions. Write your answer on the line or in the space provided.

A. Fundamentals of Written Communication

Indicate the error(s) in the statement. Then rewrite the sentence correcting the error.

1. To patients arrived at the same time.

   Error(s):_____

   New sentence: _____

2. Zac the receptionist greet the patients when they arrived.

   Error(s):_____

   New sentence: _____

3. My appointment is on August 17th 20XX.

   Error(s):_____

   New sentence: _____

4. Yesterday, Betsy and Sue work with Dr Jones.

   Error(s):_____

   New sentence: _____

5. Marie and me arrived early at the medical office

   Error(s):_____

   New sentence: _____

6. Yes i will need your new insurance card.

   Error(s):_____

   New sentence: _____

7. Thank you katie for all your hard work.

   Error(s):_____

   New sentence: _____

8. The mother father and son arrived late for there appointments.

   Error(s):_____

   New sentence: _____

9. Wear did the patient go.

   Error(s):_____

   New sentence: _____

10. There parents are talking with the provider.

   Error(s):_____

   New sentence: _____

B. Written Correspondence

1. Discuss how the medical assistant uses electronic technology in professional communication._____

   _____

   _____

   _____

2. Describe the size of the paper, margins, and line spacing used in professional letters. _____

   _____

   _____

3. What information is found in the sender's address?_____

   _____

   _____

4. What is the correct format and location for the date? _____

_____

_____

5. What is the purpose of the reference line in a professional letter? _____

_____

6. How would you compose a greeting for a professional letter to John White? _____

_____

_____

7. Where is the closing located and what are typical professional closings? _____

_____

_____

8. What are two ways a reference notation would be keyed if Jean Moore were typing a letter for Dr. Sam Mast?

_____

_____

9. Where is the reference notation placed? _____

_____

10. Describe how to add a copy notation to a letter. _____

_____

11. Name three items that should be on a continuation page. _____

_____

12. Describe the difference between closed and open punctuation in a letter. _____

_____

_____

13. Describe a full block letter format. _____

_____

_____

14. Describe the similarities and differences between the modified block letter format and the semi-block letter format.

_____

_____

_____

15. What are letter templates? _____

    _____

16. Business letters should be enclosed in standard _____ envelopes, which measure

    _____.

17. Letters and memos use the _____ orientation.

18. List the four headings used in memoranda and include the correct punctuation. _____

    _____

    _____

    _____

19. Explain why medical assistants need to know how to compose a professional email. _____

    _____

    _____

20. The following questions relate to composing professional emails.

    a. What type of greeting should be used and give an example? _____

       _____

    b. Refrain from using all capital letters. How may the reader interpret this? _____

       _____

    c. Can texting abbreviations and emoticons (emojis) be used? _____

       _____

    d. How should you end your email? _____

       _____

    e. When emailing a patient, what should occur with a copy of the sent email? _____

       _____

21. What type of information is usually on the cover sheet for a fax? _____

    _____

    _____

C. Mail

1. Describe how an automated mail processing machine reads the address on an envelope. _____

   _____

   _____

2. Describe five tips to follow when addressing mail._____

_____

_____

_____

_____

3. List four things that affect the postage rate of mail. _____

_____

4. When the healthcare facility uses Certified Mail with Return Receipt, what information does the facility get?

_____

5. Termination letters are sent by _____.

6. _____ is an optional mail service that protects against loss or damage and the cost is based on the declared value of the item.

7. _____ is an optional mail service that requires the addressee or authorized agent to verify identity when signing for the delivery.

8. _____ is an optional mail service that requires the recipient to pay for the merchandise and shipping when the package is received.

CERTIFICATION PREPARATION
Circle the correct answer.

1. Which is a word or group of words that describes a noun or pronoun?
   a. Adverb
   b. Adjective
   c. Verb
   d. Noun

2. Which needs to be capitalized?
   a. The first letter of the first word in a sentence or question
   b. The first letter of proper nouns
   c. The pronoun "I"
   d. All of the above

3. When should a comma be used?
   a. Before a coordinator (and, but, yet, nor, for, or, so) that links two main clauses
   b. To separate items in a list of three or more things
   c. After certain words (e.g., yes, no) at the start of a sentence
   d. All of the above

4. What type of software allows the user to enter demographic information, schedule appointments, maintain lists of insurance payers, perform billing tasks, and generate reports?
   a. Electronic health record (EHR)
   b. Electronic medical records (EMR)
   c. Practice management
   d. Microsoft Word and Excel

5. What includes the initials of the person who composed the letter?
   a. Enclosure notation
   b. Reference notation
   c. Copy notation
   d. Attachment notation

6. Which type of business letter format has the sender's and inside addresses left-justified and the date, closing, and signature blocks starting at the center point or right-justified?
   a. Semi-block
   b. Memo
   c. Modified block
   d. Full block

7. Which is the most commonly used mail service used for envelopes weighing up to 13 ounces, and provides delivery in 3 days or less?
   a. Priority Mail
   b. Priority Mail Express
   c. First-Class Mail
   d. Media Mail

8. Which optional mail service is used to protect expensive items, a mailing receipt is provided, and upon request an electronic verification of delivery or delivery attempt can be sent?
   a. Registered Mail
   b. Standard Insurance
   c. Certified Mail
   d. Return Receipt

9. Dr. James Smith composed a letter and Cathy Black keyed the letter. What is the correct format for the notation in the letter?
   a. cb:JS
   b. JS:cb
   c. CB:js
   d. js:CB

10. Which is *not* a header in a memo?
    a. TO
    b. FROM
    c. DEPARTMENT
    d. SUBJECT

WORKPLACE APPLICATIONS

1. Christiana Zwellen CMA (AAMA) is composing the following letters. Indicate the name that should appear in the signature block.

   a. A letter from her to the office supply company. _____

   b. A letter to Mrs. White from Dr. James Martin. _____

   c. A referral letter about a patient from Dr. James Martin to Dr. Robert Black. _____

   _____

2. When Christiana Zwellen is composing a letter for Dr. James Martin, indicate two ways she can create the reference notation.

   _____

   _____

3. Christiana needs to fold a letter for a #10 envelope. Describe how this is done. _____

   _____

   _____

INTERNET ACTIVITIES

1. Research professional email etiquette. Describe five ways you can improve your written communication with patients and professionals.

   _____

   _____

   _____

2. Research the two-letter postal abbreviations for the states. Write each address provided as it should appear on an envelope. Use only approved U.S. Postal Service standard street abbreviations and the two-letter postal abbreviation for states.

    a. Walden-Martin Family Medical Clinic, 1234 Any Street, Anytown, Alabama 14453 _____

       _____

       _____

    b. John Smith, 383 E. Center, Anytown, Nebraska 13333-2232 _____

       _____

       _____

    c. Sally Black, 39291 S. Parkway, Anytown, Wisconsin 54334-6443 _____

       _____

       _____

    d. Jeff Jones, 454 Boulevard, Anytown, Minnesota 49932-1234 _____

       _____

       _____

    e. Sam House, 599 State Highway, Anytown, Illinois 69532-1651 _____

       _____

       _____

3. Use the zip code look-up tool on www.usps.com to find the zip codes for the following cities. Write the zip code on the line to the right of the city.

    a. Chicken, AK _____

    b. Rabbit Hash, KY _____

    c. Oatmeal, TX _____

    d. Turkey, TX _____

    e. Popcorn, IN _____

    f. Toast, NC _____

    g. Corn, OK _____

    h. Cucumber, WV _____

    i. Chili, WI _____

    j. Cream, WI _____

7. Key a proper closing starting at the left margin and use the correct spelling and punctuation. Leave one blank line between the last line of the body and the closing.	10			
8. Key the signature block starting at the left margin and use the correct spelling and punctuation. Leave four blank lines between the closing and the signature block. If you are preparing the letter for a provider, you must include a reference notation.	10			
9. Spell-check and proofread the document. Check for the proper tone, grammar, punctuation, capitalization, and sentence structure. Check for proper spacing between the parts of the letter. Make any final corrections. Print the document.	5			
10. Address the envelope, using either the computer and word processing software or a pen and following the correct format.	10			
11. When using a #10 envelope, fold the letter by pulling up the bottom end until it reaches just below the inside address or two-thirds of the way up the letter. Crease at the fold. Then, fold the top of the letter down so that it is flush with the bottom fold and crease the paper.	5			
12. File a copy of the letter in the paper medical record or upload an electronic copy of the letter to the electronic health record (EHR).	5			
Total Points	100			

Comments

CAAHEP Competencies	Step(s)
V.P.8. Compose professional correspondence utilizing electronic technology	Entire procedure
ABHES Competencies	**Step(s)**
7. Administrative Procedures g. Display professionalism through written and verbal communications	Entire procedure
7.h. Perform basic computer skills	Entire procedure

Procedure 9.2 Compose a Professional Business Letter Using the Modified Block Letter Format

Name _____ Date _____ Score _____

Task: Compose a professional letter using technology. Use the modified block letter format (with the center point option). Address the envelope (if needed) and fold the letter.

Scenario: Julie Walden, MD has requested that you compose a letter to Carl C. Bowden (DOB: 04/05/1954 to let him know that his hepatitis C laboratory test was negative. If he has any questions, he should call the office. His address is 19 Beale Street, Anytown, AL 12345-1234. You are working at Walden-Martin Family Medical Clinic. The healthcare facility's address is 1234 Anystreet, Anytown, AL 12345. The phone number is 123-123-1234 and the fax number is 123-123-5678.

Equipment and Supplies:
- Patient's health record
- Computer with word processing software and printer
- Paper
- #10 envelope or window business envelope

Standard: Complete the procedure and all critical steps with a minimum score of 85% within two attempts (or as indicated by the instructor).

Scoring: Divide the points earned by the total possible points. Failure to perform a critical step, indicated by an asterisk (*), results in grade no higher than an 84% (or as indicated by the instructor).

Steps:	Point Value	Attempt 1	Attempt 2
1. Obtain the intended recipient's contact information and determine the message you want to convey. Using the computer and word processing software, compose the letter using the modified block letter format. Use 1-inch margins on all four sides, portrait orientation, and use single line spacing throughout the letter. Use an easy-to-read font (e.g., Times New Roman or Calibri), in a 10- or 12-point size.	5		
2. Create a letterhead in the header of the document. Include the clinic's name, street address or post office box, city, state, and ZIP code.	10		
3. Key (type) the date starting at the center point of the document. Have one blank line between the date line and the last line of the letterhead.	10		
4. Key the inside address starting at the left margin and use the correct spelling and punctuation. Leave one to nine blank lines between the date and the inside address, to center the body of the letter on the page. If using a window business envelope, adjust the address position to fit the window.	10*		
5. Key the salutation starting at the left margin and use the correct spelling and punctuation. Leave one blank line between the inside address and the salutation.	10		

		Points		
6.	Use your critical thinking skills to compose a concise, accurate message. Type the message in the body of the letter starting at the left margin. Leave one blank line between the salutation and the first line of the body and then between each paragraph of the body. The message should be clear, concise, and professional. Use proper grammar, punctuation, capitalization, and sentence structure.	10		
7.	Key a proper closing starting at the center point of the document. Use the correct spelling and punctuation. Leave one blank line between the last line of the body and the closing.	10		
8.	Key the signature block starting at the center point of the document. Use the correct spelling and punctuation. Leave four blank lines between the closing and the signature block. If you are preparing the letter for a provider, you must include a reference notation.	10		
9.	Spell-check and proofread the document. Check for the proper tone, grammar, punctuation, capitalization, and sentence structure. Check for proper spacing between the parts of the letter. Make any final corrections. Print the document. If needed, address the envelope, using either the computer and word processing software or a pen and following the correct format.	10		
10.	When using a #10 envelope, fold the letter by pulling up the bottom end until it reaches just below the inside address or two-thirds of the way up the letter. Crease at the fold. Then, fold the top of the letter down so that it is flush with the bottom fold and crease the paper. For window business envelopes, have the letter's print side facing up and place the envelope over the top third of the letter. Fold the bottom edge of the paper up to the bottom edge of the envelope and crease at the fold. Then, remove the envelope and flip the letter over and fold the top of the letter down to the prior crease line and crease at the fold. Place the letter in the envelope so that the recipient's address shows through the window.	10		
11.	File a copy of the letter in the paper medical record or upload an electronic copy of the letter to the electronic health record (EHR).	5		
	Total Points	**100**		

Comments

CAAHEP Competencies	Step(s)
V.P.8. Compose professional correspondence utilizing electronic technology	Entire procedure
ABHES Competencies	**Step(s)**
7. Administrative Procedures g. Display professionalism through written and verbal communications	Entire procedure
7.h. Perform basic computer skills	Entire procedure

Procedure 9.3   Compose a Professional Business Letter Using the Semi-Block Letter Format

Name _____   Date _____   Score _____

Task: Compose a professional letter using technology. Use the semi-block letter format (with the right justified option). Address the envelope and fold the letter.

Scenario: Julie Walden MD has requested that you compose a letter to Amma Patel to let her know that her thyroid test was normal, but her vitamin D level was low. Dr. Walden would like Amma to take 15 mcg of vitamin D each morning. She can purchase this over the counter. She needs to have her vitamin D rechecked in 6 months. She can call to schedule the blood test closer to that time. If she has any questions, she should call the office. Her address is 1346 Charity Lane, Anytown, AL 12345-1234. You are working at Walden-Martin Family Medical Clinic. The healthcare facility's address is 1234 Anystreet, Anytown, AL 12345. The phone number is 123-123-1234 and the fax number is 123-123-5678.

Equipment and Supplies:
- Patient's health record
- Computer with word processing software and printer
- Paper
- #10 envelope or #6¾ envelope

Standard: Complete the procedure and all critical steps with a minimum score of 85% within two attempts (or as indicated by the instructor).

Scoring: Divide the points earned by the total possible points. Failure to perform a critical step, indicated by an asterisk (*), results in grade no higher than an 84% (or as indicated by the instructor).

Steps:	Point Value	Attempt 1	Attempt 2
1. Obtain the intended recipient's contact information and determine the message you want to convey. Using the computer and word processing software, compose the letter using the semi-block letter format. Use 1-inch margins on all four sides, portrait orientation, and use single line spacing throughout the letter. Use an easy-to-read font (e.g., Times New Roman or Calibri), in a 10- or 12-point size.	5		
2. Create a letterhead in the header of the document. Include the clinic's name, street address or post office box, city, state, and ZIP code.	10		
3. Right justify and key (type) the date. Have one blank line between the date line and the last line of the letterhead.	10		
4. Key the inside address starting at the left margin and use the correct spelling and punctuation. Leave one to nine blank lines between the date and the inside address, to center the body of the letter on the page.	10*		
5. Key the salutation starting at the left margin and use the correct spelling and punctuation. Leave one blank line between the inside address and the salutation.	10		

6.	Use your critical thinking skills to compose a concise, accurate message. Type the message in the body of the letter starting at the left margin. Leave one blank line between the salutation and the first line of the body and then between each paragraph of the body. Each paragraph should be indented five spaces. The message should be clear, concise, and professional. Use proper grammar, punctuation, capitalization, and sentence structure.	10		
7.	Right justify and key a proper closing. Use the correct spelling and punctuation. Leave one blank line between the last line of the body and the closing.	10		
8.	Right justify and key the signature block. Use the correct spelling and punctuation. Leave four blank lines between the closing and the signature block. If you are preparing the letter for a provider, you must include a reference notation.	10		
9.	Spell-check and proofread the document. Check for the proper tone, grammar, punctuation, capitalization, and sentence structure. Check for proper spacing between the parts of the letter. Make any final corrections. Print the document.	5		
10.	Address the envelope, using either the computer and word processing software or a pen and following the correct format.	10		
11.	When using a #10 envelope, fold the letter by pulling up the bottom end until it reaches just below the inside address or two-thirds of the way up the letter. Crease at the fold. Then, fold the top of the letter down so that it is flush with the bottom fold and crease the paper. When using a #6¾ envelope, pull the bottom edge of the letter up until it is ½ inch from the top edge of the document and crease at the fold. Bring the right edge two-thirds of the way across the width of the document and crease the paper. Then bring the left edge to the right edge and crease at the fold. Flip the document so the left edge is on the bottom and insert the letter into the envelope.	5		
12.	File a copy of the letter in the paper medical record or upload an electronic copy of the letter to the electronic health record (EHR).	5		
	Total Points	100		

Comments

CAAHEP Competencies	Step(s)
V.P.8. Compose professional correspondence utilizing electronic technology	Entire procedure
ABHES Competencies	**Step(s)**
7. Administrative Procedures g. Display professionalism through written and verbal communications	Entire procedure
7.h. Perform basic computer skills	Entire procedure

Procedure 9.4   Compose a Memorandum

Name _____   Date _____   Score _____

Task: Compose a professional memorandum.

Scenario: You are asked by the supervisor to compose a memo that can be posted in the department. You are to remind the staff about the department meeting next Tuesday at noon in the conference room. Staff can bring their lunches and beverages will be provided.

Equipment and Supplies:
- Computer with word processing software and printer
- Paper

Standard: Complete the procedure and all critical steps with a minimum score of 85% within two attempts (or as indicated by the instructor).

Scoring: Divide the points earned by the total possible points. Failure to perform a critical step, indicated by an asterisk (*), results in grade no higher than an 84% (or as indicated by the instructor).

Steps:	Point Value	Attempt 1	Attempt 2
1. Determine the message you want to convey. Using the computer and word processing software, compose the memo. Use 1-inch margins on all four sides, portrait orientation, and use single line spacing throughout the memo. Use an easy-to-read font (e.g., Times New Roman or Calibri), in a 10- or 12-point size.	15		
2. Left justify the headers and use boldface and capital letters, followed by a colon. Headers include TO, FROM, DATE, and SUBJECT. Leave one blank line between each header.	15		
3. Key (type) the information following the headers in regular font, using a mix of capital and lowercase letters. Using the tab tool, align the information vertically down the page. Key (type) the date as indicated for professional letters.	15		
4. Add a centered black line between the headers and the body (optional). Leave two to three blank lines between the headers and the body of the memo.	15		
5. Key the message in the body of the memo. Left justify the content in the body and use single line spacing. Use proper grammar and correct spelling and punctuation. With multiple paragraphs, skip a single line between paragraphs.	15		
6. The content of the message in the body of the memo is written clearly, concisely, and accurately. Add special notations as needed.	15		
7. Spell-check and proofread the document. Check for the proper tone, grammar, punctuation, capitalization, and sentence structure. Check for proper spacing between the parts of the memo. Make any final corrections. Print the document.	10		
Total Points	100		

Comments

CAAHEP Competencies	Step(s)
V.P.8. Compose professional correspondence utilizing electronic technology	Entire procedure
ABHES Competencies	**Step(s)**
7. Administrative Procedures g. Display professionalism through written and verbal communications	Entire procedure
7.h. Perform basic computer skills	Entire procedure

Procedure 9.5   Compose a Professional Email

Name _____   Date _____   Score _____

Task: Compose a professional email that conveys the message to the reader clearly, concisely, and accurately.

Scenario: Aaron Jackson (DOB: 10/17/2011) has an appointment at 11 AM next Thursday. Send his guardian an appointment reminder via email. Aaron will be seeing David Kahn, M.D. The guardian should bring in any medications Aaron is currently taking. You are working at Walden-Martin Family Medical Clinic. The healthcare facility's address is: 1234 Anystreet, Anytown, AL 12345. The phone number is 123-123-1234 and the fax number is 123-123-5678. Your instructor will supply you with the guardian's name and email address.

Equipment and Supplies:
- Patient's health record
- Computer with email software

Standard: Complete the procedure and all critical steps with a minimum score of 85% within two attempts (or as indicated by the instructor).

Scoring: Divide the points earned by the total possible points. Failure to perform a critical step, indicated by an asterisk (*), results in grade no higher than an 84% (or as indicated by the instructor).

Steps:	Point Value	Attempt 1	Attempt 2
1. Obtain the intended recipient's contact information and determine the message you want to convey.	5		
2. Using the computer and email software, key (type) in the recipient's email address. If the email has two recipients, use a semicolon (;) after the name of the first recipient. Double-check the email addresses for accuracy.	5*		
3. Key in a subject, keeping it simple but focused on the contents of the email.	10		
4. Key a formal greeting, using correct punctuation.	10		
5. Key the message in the body of the email using proper grammar, punctuation, capitalization, and sentence structure. Avoid abbreviations. The message should be clear, concise, and professional.	20		
6. Finish the email with closing remarks.	10		
7. Key a closing, followed by your name and title on the next line. Include the clinic's name and contact information below your name.	10		
8. Spell-check and proofread the email. Check for proper tone, grammar, punctuation, capitalization, and sentence structure. Check for proper spacing between the parts of the email.	10		
9. Make any final revisions, select any features to apply to the email, and then send it.	10		
10. Print a copy of the email to be filed in the paper medical record or upload an electronic copy of the email to the patient's electronic health record (EHR).	10		
Total Points	100		

Comments

CAAHEP Competencies	Step(s)
V.P.8. Compose professional correspondence utilizing electronic technology	Entire procedure
ABHES Competencies	**Step(s)**
7. Administrative Procedures g. Display professionalism through written and verbal communications	Entire procedure
7.h. Perform basic computer skills	Entire procedure

Procedure 9.6 Complete a Fax Cover Sheet

Name _____ Date _____ Score _____

Task: Complete a fax cover sheet clearly and accurately.

Scenario: Lisa Parker, mother of Johnny Parker (DOB: 06/15/2010) requested his immunization history be sent to Anytown School, attention: Susie Payne. The school's phone number is 123-123-5784 and the fax number will be supplied by your instructor. The release of medical records has been completed and signed by Lisa, Johnny's guardian/mother. Your phone number is the main clinic number listed on the header of the fax cover sheet.

Equipment and Supplies:
- Document to be faxed (optional)
- Fax machine and fax number (optional)
- Pen
- Fax cover sheet (Work Product 9.1, HIPAA-Compliant Fax Cover Sheet)

Standard: Complete the procedure and all critical steps with a minimum score of 85% within two attempts (or as indicated by the instructor).

Scoring: Divide the points earned by the total possible points. Failure to perform a critical step, indicated by an asterisk (*), results in grade no higher than an 84% (or as indicated by the instructor).

Steps:	Point Value	Attempt 1	Attempt 2
1. Using a pen and the fax cover sheet, clearly and accurately write your name, phone number, and the date.	20		
2. Clearly and accurately write the name of the person receiving the fax. Also include the company, fax number, and the phone number.	20		
3. Write the number of pages. The cover sheet must be counted in the total.	20		
4. Complete Re: by indicating the subject of the fax. Be general with the subject and refrain from including anything confidential.	20		
5. Proofread the fax cover sheet. Verify the name, agency, and contact information of the recipient. Verify the document(s) being sent are correct. Organize the documents so the coversheet is on top and fax to the recipient (optional).	20		
Total Points	100		

Comments

ABHES Competencies	Step(s)
7. Administrative Procedures g. Display professionalism through written and verbal communications	Entire procedure

Work Product 9.1   HIPAA-Compliant Fax Cover Sheet

To be used with Procedure 9.6.

Name _____   Date _____   Score _____

WALDEN-MARTIN
FAMILY MEDICAL CLINIC
1234 ANYSTREET | ANYTOWN, ANYSTATE 12345
PHONE 123-123-1234 | FAX 123-123-5678

Fax

To: _____	From: _____
Company: _____	Phone: _____
Fax: _____	Date: _____
Phone: _____	
Pages: _____	
Re: _____	

CONFIDENTIAL NOTICE

The material enclosed with this facsimile transmission is confidential and private. The material is the property of the sender and some or all of the information may be protected by the Health Insurance Portability & Accountability Act (HIPAA). This information is intended exclusively for the addressed person or agency indicated above. If you are not the intended individual or entity of this information, you are hereby notified that any use, duplication, circulation, or transmission of the information is strictly prohibited under state and federal law. Please notify the sender immediate using the telephone number indicated above.

Telephone Techniques

CAAHEP	Assessments
V.P.6. Demonstrate professional telephone techniques	Procedure 10.1
V.P.7. Document telephone messages accurately	Procedure 10.2
V.P.11. Report relevant information concisely and accurately	Procedure 10.2

ABHES	Assessments
7. Administrative Procedures g. Display professionalism through written and verbal communications	Procedure 10.1, 10.2

VOCABULARY REVIEW

Using the word pool on the right, find the correct word to match the definition. Write the word on the line after the definition.

Group A

1. A commercial service that answers telephone calls for its clients

   _____

2. An unexpected, life-threatening situation that requires immediate action _____

3. A business telephone system that allows for more than one telephone line _____

4. A feature that states who the caller is and displays the telephone numbers of incoming calls made to a particular line

   _____

5. The depth of a tone or sound; a distinctive quality of sound

   _____

6. A telephone feature that allows calls made to one number to be sent to another specified number _____

7. An applied science concerned with designing and arranging things needed to do your job in an efficient and safe way

   _____

8. An individual or company that supplies medical care and services to a patient or the public _____

9. A telephone with a loudspeaker and a microphone; it can be used without having to pick up and hold the handset

   _____

10. A telephone function in which a selected stored number can be dialed by pressing only one key _____

11. An electronic system that allows messages from telephone callers to be recorded and stored _____

12. A two-way communication system with a microphone and loudspeaker at each station; often a feature of business telephones

    _____

Word Pool
- multiple line telephone system
- ergonomics
- speakerphone
- caller ID
- voice mail
- emergency
- call forwarding
- answering service
- intercom
- provider
- speed dialing
- pitch

Group B

1. Ability to communicate effectively in two languages
   _____

2. A physician or other healthcare provider who enters into a contract with a specific insurance company or program and by doing so agrees to abide by certain rules and regulations set forth by that third-party payer _____

3. A set dollar amount that the patient must pay for each visit
   _____

4. A system that distributes incoming calls to a specific group or person based on customer need; for example, the customer presses 1 for appointments, 2 for billing questions, and so on
   _____

5. A succession of syllables, words, or sentences spoken in an unvaried key or pitch _____

6. The use of articulate, clear sounds when speaking
   _____

7. The quality of having a sense of what to do or say to maintain good relations with others or to prevent offense
   _____

8. The vocabulary of a particular profession as opposed to common, everyday terms _____

9. A system for examining and separating into different groups; in the healthcare facility, it means determining the severity of illness that patients experience and prioritizing appointments based on that severity _____

10. The process of assigning degrees of urgency to patients' conditions _____

11. An acute situation that requires immediate attention but is not life-threatening _____

12. The medical abbreviation for the Latin term *statum*, meaning immediately; at this moment _____

Word Pool

- monotone
- enunciation
- tactful
- jargon
- screen
- triage
- urgent
- copayment (copay)
- participating provider
- STAT
- bilingual
- automatic call routing

SKILLS AND CONCEPTS

Answer the following questions. Write your answer on the line or in the space provided.

A. Telephone Equipment

1. Give an example of when the following telephone features would be used.

   Speakerphone: _____

   _____

   _____

   _____

   _____

Conference calls: _____

_____

_____

_____

_____

Voice mail: _____

_____

_____

_____

_____

Call forwarding: _____

_____

_____

_____

_____

Intercom: _____

_____

_____

_____

_____

B. Telephone Equipment Needs of a Healthcare Facility

1. Describe the minimum number of telephone lines needed in a healthcare facility._____

_____

_____

C. Effective Use of the Telephone

1. List three things involved in active listening.

    a. _____

    b. _____

    c. _____

2. If you are speaking clearly and distinctly, you are using good _____.

3. It is important to make sure that our patients understand what we are saying to them. In healthcare, medical terminology or _____ can make things more difficult for patients to understand.

D. Managing Telephone Calls

1. List the supplies needed to be prepared to answer incoming telephone calls. _____

_____

_____

_____

_____

2. How should a second incoming call be handled when you are already answering another call?

_____

_____

_____

_____

3. How should a caller who refuses to identify him- or herself be handled? _____

_____

_____

_____

_____

_____

4. List the conditions and/or symptoms that would be considered an emergency call. _____

_____

_____

_____

_____

5. What questions should be asked of the patient who calls the healthcare facility to give the provider the information that he or she needs?

_____

_____

_____

_____

E. Typical Incoming Calls

1. When a patient calls requesting a medication refill, what information is needed? _____

   _____

   _____

   _____

   _____

   _____

2. How should requests for directions be handled? _____

   _____

   _____

   _____

3. When a patient calls and asks for a referral to another provider, what should the medical assistant do?

   _____

   _____

   _____

   _____

   _____

F. Special Incoming Calls

1. If a patient refuses to discuss his or her symptoms over the phone with the medical assistant and the provider is not able to take the call, what should the medical assistant suggest the patient do?

   _____

   _____

2. What is the best policy when a patient calls for test results that are abnormal?_____

   _____

   _____

3. What documentation should be in place before a medical assistant can give information to a third party?

   _____

   _____

4. How should a caller with a complaint be handled? _____

_____

_____

_____

G. Handling Difficult Calls
Indicate how you would handle the following calls.

1. Angry callers:_____

_____

_____

_____

_____

2. Aggressive callers: _____

_____

_____

_____

_____

3. Unauthorized inquiry calls:_____

_____

_____

_____

_____

4. Sales calls:_____

_____

_____

_____

_____

5. Callers who speak foreign languages or have heavy accents: _____

_____

_____

_____

_____

H. Typical Outgoing Calls

1. Use Figure 10.4 in the textbook to answer the following questions.

    a. You are in the Central time zone and need to call an insurance carrier in the Pacific time zone. It is 9:00 AM in your location. What time is it in the Pacific time zone?

    _____

    b. You are in the Pacific time zone and your provider has asked you to contact another provider in the Eastern time zone. It is 10:00 AM in your time zone. What time is it in the Eastern time zone?

    _____

    c. You are in the Eastern time zone and need to contact a patient who is vacationing in the Mountain time zone. It is 3:00 PM in your time zone. What time is it in the Mountain time zone?

    _____

I. Using Directory Assistance

1. List options for locating a telephone number. _____

_____

_____

_____

_____

J. Telephone Services

1. Explain the difference between an answering machine and answering service. _____

_____

_____

_____

_____

CERTIFICATION PREPARATION

Circle the correct answer.

1. Which best describes the primary goal of "screening" telephone calls?
   a. Preventing calls from reaching the provider
   b. Handling calls at the lowest level possible
   c. Selecting which calls should be forwarded to which staff members through an understanding of the purpose of the call
   d. Determining whether the calls are emergencies

2. Active listening involves
   a. giving the same attention to a person on the telephone as would be given to a person face to face.
   b. concentrating on the conversation at hand.
   c. discovering vital information.
   d. all of the above.

3. The medical assistant should be extremely careful when using a speakerphone because
   a. the service is expensive.
   b. it is distracting.
   c. the call can be traced.
   d. confidentiality can be violated.

4. Which term would be considered jargon?
   a. Encephalalgia
   b. Rash
   c. Dizziness
   d. Headache

5. The medical assistant may help an angry caller calm down by
   a. getting angry in return.
   b. speaking in a lower tone of voice.
   c. referring the situation to the office manager immediately.
   d. calling the provider into the situation.

6. If your office is in New York and you need to contact a supplier in Seattle, which New York time would be the earliest that you should call to place an order, assuming that the supplier opens at 8 AM?
   a. 8:00 AM
   b. 9:00 AM
   c. 10:00 AM
   d. 11:00 AM

7. Which types of calls should be limited in the professional setting?
   a. Local
   b. Long distance
   c. Toll free
   d. Personal

8. Enunciation is
   a. the choice of words.
   b. the highness or lowness of sound.
   c. articulation of clear sounds.
   d. a change in pitch.

9. Which is *not* required when a telephone message is taken?
   a. The caller's name and phone number
   b. The time and date
   c. The name of the person to whom the call is directed
   d. The caller's account number

10. When placing callers on hold, how often should you check back to make sure the caller still wants to remain on hold?
    a. No longer than 1 minute
    b. Every 2 minutes
    c. Until time is available to talk
    d. It is not necessary to check back; patients will hold until you return to the call

WORKPLACE APPLICATIONS

1. Mr. Ken Thomas calls to get his prescription for Ambien refilled. His pharmacy is Wolfe Drug, and the drugstore phone number is 214-555-4523. Mr. Thomas is allergic to penicillin. His phone number is 214-555-2377. Mr. Thomas' message was received on July 23 at 10:15 AM.

   a. Who should receive this message? _____

   _____

   b. Questions to ask the patient: _____

   _____

   _____

   c. What action should be taken after speaking with the patient?_____

   _____

   _____

   _____

   _____

2. Message retrieved from the answering machine, "This is Sarah at AnyTown Lab with a STAT laboratory report. It is 9:35 AM on November 16. The patient's name is Noemi Rodriguez, date of birth November 4, 1971 and her WBC count is 18,000. Please notify Dr. Walden immediately. The laboratory phone number is 800-555-3333 and my extension is 255. If she has any questions, please have her give me a call. Thanks."

   a. Who should receive this message? _____

   _____

   b. Questions to ask Sarah:_____

   _____

   _____

   c. What action should be taken? _____

   _____

   _____

   _____

   _____

   _____

3. Denise has been the receptionist for a moderately large clinic for the past 3 months. She replaced Dorothy, who retired. Denise has been overwhelmed with the calls to the clinic, and the office manager has spoken to her twice about missing calls. Denise insists that she is constantly on the phone answering and transferring calls. She is beginning to lose faith in herself, but as she considers why she is failing at her job, she realizes that two new physicians have joined the practice since Dorothy left, and numerous calls come to the clinic for those two providers. Denise wants to suggest to the office manager that perhaps the time has come for a second receptionist, but she is unsure how to broach the subject. How can Denise begin her conversation with the office manager? What should she not do or say?

_____

_____

_____

_____

_____

_____

INTERNET ACTIVITIES

1. Using online resources, locate the following telephone numbers for your city or community.

    a. Nonemergency number for the police department _____

    b. Local social security office _____

    c. American Red Cross office _____

    d. Acute care hospital _____

    e. Meals on Wheels _____

    f. American Cancer Society _____

    g. Local senior center _____

    h. Local food bank _____

    i. Poison control _____

    j. Local child protective services _____

Procedure 10.1   Demonstrate Professional Telephone Techniques

Name _____ Date _____ Score _____

Task: To answer the telephone in a provider's office in a professional manner and respond to a request for action.

Scenario: Charles Johnson, DOB 3/3/1958, an established patient of Dr. Martin, has called to schedule an appointment to have his blood pressure checked. This will be a follow-up appointment that is 15 minutes long. He is requesting that the appointment be on a Friday during his lunchtime between 11:00 and 12:00.

Equipment and Supplies:
- Telephone
- Pen or pencil
- Computer
- Notepad

Standard: Complete the procedure and all critical steps in _____ minutes with a minimum score of 85% within two attempts (*or as indicated by the instructor*).

Scoring: Divide the points earned by the total possible points. Failure to perform a critical step, indicated by an asterisk (*), results in grade no higher than an 84% (*or as indicated by the instructor*).

Time: Began_____ Ended_____ Total minutes: _____

Steps:	Point Value	Attempt 1	Attempt 2
1. Demonstrate telephone techniques by answering the telephone by the third ring.	10		
2. Speak distinctly with a pleasant tone and expression, at a moderate rate, and with sufficient volume for the person to understand every word.	15*		
3. Identify the office and/or provider and yourself.	10		
4. Verify the identity of the caller, and if using an electronic health record, bring the patient's health record to the active screen of the computer.	15*		
5. Screen the call if necessary.	10		
6. Apply active listening skills to assess whether the caller is distressed or agitated and to determine the concern to be addressed.	10*		
7. Determine the needs of the caller and provide the requested information or service if possible. Provide the caller with excellent customer service. Be as helpful as possible. Check the appointment schedule and determine the first Friday that would have an open appointment between 11:00 and 12:00	10		
8. Obtain sufficient patient information to schedule the appointment, including the patient's full name, DOB, insurance information, and preferred contact method. Repeat the date and time of the appointment to ensure that the patient has the correct information.	10		
9. Terminate the call in a pleasant manner and replace the receiver gently, always allowing the caller to hang up first.	10		
Total Points	100		

Comments

CAAHEP Competencies	Step(s)
V.P.6. Demonstrate professional telephone techniques	Entire procedure
ABHES Competencies	**Step(s)**
7. Administrative Procedures g. Display professionalism through written and verbal communications	Entire procedure

Procedure 10.2   Document Telephone Messages and Report Relevant Information Concisely and Accurately

Name _____ Date _____ Score _____

Tasks: To take an accurate telephone message and follow up on the requests made by the caller.

Scenario: Norma Washington, DOB 8/1/1944, an established patient of Dr. Martin, has called to report her blood pressure readings that she has been taking at home. Dr. Martin had made a recent change in her medication and wanted her to monitor her BP at home for 3 days and call in with the results. She has taken her blood pressure in the morning and in the evening for the past 3 days, with the following results:
- Day 1: 144/92 in the AM, 156/94 in the PM
- Day 2: 136/84 in the AM, 142/86 in the PM
- Day 3: 132/80 in the AM, 138/82 in the PM

Equipment and Supplies:
- Telephone
- Computer or message pad
- Pen or pencil
- Health record

Standard: Complete the procedure and all critical steps in _____ minutes with a minimum score of 85% within two attempts (*or as indicated by the instructor*).

Scoring: Divide the points earned by the total possible points. Failure to perform a critical step, indicated by an asterisk (*), results in grade no higher than an 84% (*or as indicated by the instructor*).

Time: Began _____ Ended _____ Total minutes: _____

Steps:	Point Value	Attempt 1	Attempt 2
1. Demonstrate telephone techniques by answering the telephone using the guidelines in Procedure 10.1.	15		
2. Using a message pad or the computer, take the phone message (either on paper or by data entry into the computer) and obtain the following information: • Name of the person to whom the call is directed • Name of the person calling • Caller's telephone number • Reason for the call • Action to be taken • Date and time of the call • Initials of the person taking the call	15*		
3. Apply active listening skills and repeat the information back to the caller after recording the message.	10		
4. End the call and wait for the caller to hang up first.	10		
5. Document the telephone call with all pertinent information in the patient's health record.	10*		
6. Deliver the phone message to the appropriate person.	10		

7.	Follow up on important messages.	**10**		
8.	If using paper messaging, keep old message books for future reference. Carbonless copies allow the facility to keep a permanent record of phone messages. If using an electronic system, the message will be saved to the patient's record automatically.	**10**		
9.	File pertinent phone messages in the patient's health record. Make sure the computer record is closed after the documentation has been done.	**10**		
	Total Points	**100**		

Comments

CAAHEP Competencies	Step(s)
V.P.6. Demonstrate professional telephone techniques	1, 3, 4
V.P.7. Document telephone messages accurately	2, 5
ABHES Competencies	**Step(s)**
7. Administrative Procedures g. Display professionalism through written and verbal communications	Entire procedure

Scheduling Appointments and Patient Processing

CAAHEP	Assessments
VI.C.1. Identify different types of appointment scheduling methods	Skills and Concepts – C. 1-6
VI.C.2.a. Identify advantages and disadvantages of the following appointment systems: manual	Skills and Concepts – C. 2
VI.C.2.b. Identify advantages and disadvantages of the following appointment systems: electronic	Skills and Concepts – C. 3
VI.C.3. Identify critical information required for scheduling patient procedures	Skills and Concepts – G. 1
VI.P.1. Manage appointment schedule using established priorities	Procedure 11.1, 11.2, 11.4
VI.P.2. Schedule a patient procedure	Procedure 11.5
VI.A.1. Display sensitivity when managing appointments	Procedure 11.2, 11.4, 11.5
VII.P.3. Obtain accurate patient billing information	Procedure 11.2
V.P.4.a. Coach patients regarding: office policies	Procedure 11.3
ABHES	**Assessments**
7. Administrative Procedures e. Apply scheduling principles	Procedure 11.1, 11.2, 11.4, 11.5

VOCABULARY REVIEW

Using the word pool on the right, find the correct word to match the definition. Write the word on the line after the definition.

Group A

1. Documentation in the medical record to track the patient's condition and progress _____

2. Space of time between events _____

3. An unexpected event that throws a plan into disorder; an interruption that prevents a system or process from continuing as usual or as expected _____

4. Skilled as a result of training or practice _____

5. A rule that controls how something should be done; guidelines or boundaries _____

6. An appointment type used when a patient needs to see the provider after a condition should have been resolved or to monitor an ongoing condition _____

7. The environment where something is created or takes shape; a base on which to build _____

8. Statistical data of a population; in healthcare this includes patient name, address, date of birth, employment, and other details _____

9. A type of software that allows the user to enter demographic information, schedule appointments, maintain lists of insurance payers, perform billing tasks, and generate reports _____

10. Essential; being an indispensable part of a whole _____

Word Pool
- parameters
- demographics
- integral
- intervals
- matrix
- follow-up appointment
- proficiency
- practice management software
- progress notes
- disruption

Group B

1. A means of achieving a particular end, as in a situation requiring urgency or caution _____

2. The process of confirming health insurance coverage for the patient _____

3. A written document describing the healthcare facility's privacy practices _____

4. A system for examining and separating into different groups; in the healthcare facility, it means determining the severity of illness that patients experience and prioritizing appointments based on that severity _____

5. The process of determining if a procedure or service is covered by the insurance plan and what the reimbursement is for that procedure or service _____

6. To sort out and classify the injured; used in the military and in emergency settings to determine the priority of a patient to be treated _____

7. A patient who has been treated previously by the healthcare provider within the past 3 years _____

8. A secure online website that gives patients 24-hour access to personal health information using a username and password _____

9. When a patient fails to keep an appointment without giving advance notice _____

10. The process of determining if a procedure or service is covered by the insurance plan and what the reimbursement is for that procedure or service _____

Word Pool
- Notice of Privacy Practices
- preauthorization
- precertification
- established patients
- screening
- no-show
- expediency
- triage
- patient portal
- verification of eligibility

ABBREVIATIONS

Write out what each of the following abbreviations stands for.

1. ECG _____

2. NPP _____

3. MRI _____

4. CT _____

5. EMT _____

6. EHR _____

7. HIPAA _____

8. CDC _____

SKILLS AND CONCEPTS

Answer the following questions. Write your answer on the line or in the space provided.

Scheduling Appointments

A. Establishing the Appointment Schedule

1. When developing an appointment schedule, _____ and _____ must be considered.

2. _____ information includes the patient's address, insurance information, and email address.

B. Creating the Appointment Matrix

1. Time would be blocked out in the schedule for what four reasons when setting up the appointment matrix?

    a. _____

    b. _____

    c. _____

    d. _____

2. How can the medical assistant handle a provider who habitually spends more than the allotted time with patients?

    _____

    _____

    _____

    _____

3. Using the appointment schedule page that follows, schedule these appointments, blocking out the appropriate amount of time:

    Recheck appointment   15 minutes

    Complete physical examination (PE)   45 minutes

    a. Jana Green; recheck appointment, prefers Wednesdays
    b. Pedro Gomez; complete physical examination, prefers Tuesdays
    c. Truong Tran; recheck, prefers Thursdays after 9:00 AM
    d. Walter Biller; complete physical examination, prefers Mondays as early as possible
    e. Reuven Ahmad; complete physical examination, prefers Fridays

	Monday	Tuesday	Wednesday	Thursday	Friday
8:00					
8:15					
8:30					
8:45					
9:00					
9:15					
9:30					
9:45					
10:00					

C. Methods of Scheduling Appointments

1. Identify the different scheduling methods._____

_____

_____

2. Identify the advantages and disadvantages of a manual appointment system._____

_____

_____

_____

_____

_____

_____

3. Identify advantages and disadvantages of an electronic appointment system. _____

_____

_____

_____

_____

_____

_____

D. Types of Appointment Scheduling

Briefly describe each type of scheduling and list one advantage and one disadvantage of each.

1. Time-specified (stream) scheduling_____

    _____

    _____

    _____

    _____

    _____

    _____

2. Open office hours _____

    _____

    _____

    _____

    _____

    _____

    _____

3. Wave scheduling_____

    _____

    _____

    _____

    _____

    _____

    _____

4. Modified wave scheduling _____

    _____

    _____

    _____

    _____

    _____

    _____

5. Double booking_____

_____

_____

_____

_____

_____

6. Grouping procedures_____

_____

_____

_____

_____

_____

_____

E. Telephone Scheduling

1. When scheduling an appointment over the telephone, what options are available to remind patients of the appointment?

_____

F. Scheduling Appointments for New Patients

1. To determine how much time to allow for an appointment, the medical assistant needs to obtain information about the _____.

2. New patients should be asked to arrive _____ minutes early to complete necessary paperwork.

3. An ideal tool to provide new patients with information is a(n) _____.

G. Scheduling Other Types of Appointments

1. Identify critical information required for scheduling patient procedures. _____

_____

_____

_____

_____

_____

2. Identify the special requests that a provider may have for inpatient surgeries. _____

_____

_____

_____

_____

H. Special Circumstances

1. What is the difference between an emergency appointment and an urgent appointment? _____

_____

_____

_____

_____

2. How does the medical assistant handle a patient who arrives at the clinic to see the provider but does not have an appointment?

_____

_____

_____

_____

I. Increasing Appointment Show Rates
Practice completing appointment reminder cards on the forms provided. Students should be able to fill out the appointment cards with the information provided without difficulty.

1. Tai Yan has an appointment for August 23, 20XX, at 3:00 PM with Dr. Martin.

WALDEN-MARTIN
FAMILY MEDICAL CLINIC
1234 ANYSTREET I ANYTOWN, ANYSTATE 12345
PHONE 123-123-1234 I FAX 123-123-5678

_____

has an appointment on   provider

_____

date   time

Please telephone one day in advance if you will be unable to keep the appointment

---

2. Diego Lopez has an appointment for May 1, 20XX, at 9:00 AM with Dr. Walden.

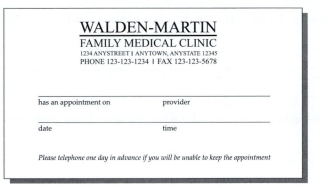

WALDEN-MARTIN
FAMILY MEDICAL CLINIC
1234 ANYSTREET I ANYTOWN, ANYSTATE 12345
PHONE 123-123-1234 I FAX 123-123-5678

_____   _____
has an appointment on   provider

_____   _____
date   time

Please telephone one day in advance if you will be unable to keep the appointment

3. Julia Berkley has an appointment for June 13, 20XX, at 11:45 AM with Dr. Walden.

WALDEN-MARTIN
FAMILY MEDICAL CLINIC
1234 ANYSTREET I ANYTOWN, ANYSTATE 12345
PHONE 123-123-1234 I FAX 123-123-5678

_____   _____
has an appointment on   provider

_____   _____
date   time

Please telephone one day in advance if you will be unable to keep the appointment

4. Monique Jones has an appointment for September 12, 20XX, at 2:40 PM with Jean Burke, N.P.

WALDEN-MARTIN
FAMILY MEDICAL CLINIC
1234 ANYSTREET I ANYTOWN, ANYSTATE 12345
PHONE 123-123-1234 I FAX 123-123-5678

_____   _____
has an appointment on   provider

_____   _____
date   time

Please telephone one day in advance if you will be unable to keep the appointment

5. Ken Thomas has an appointment for December 15, 20XX, at 4:30 PM with Dr. Martin.

WALDEN-MARTIN
FAMILY MEDICAL CLINIC
1234 ANYSTREET I ANYTOWN, ANYSTATE 12345
PHONE 123-123-1234 I FAX 123-123-5678

_____   _____
has an appointment on   provider

_____   _____
date   time

Please telephone one day in advance if you will be unable to keep the appointment

Patient Processing Tasks

1. When screening patients at the reception desk, what patient conditions require immediate action by the medical assistant?

   _____

   _____

2. What action should the medical assistant take when patients have emergent conditions? _____

   _____

   _____

   _____

3. If a medical assistant is unable to greet a patient at the reception desk, what actions can help acknowledge the person?

   _____

   _____

4. List six features of a HIPAA-appropriate sign-in register._____

   _____

   _____

   _____

   _____

   _____

   _____

5. List three features that would cause a HIPAA violation with sign-in registers._____

   _____

   _____

   _____

   _____

6. How does a medical assistant take steps to protect other patients in the reception area? _____

   _____

   _____

   _____

   _____

7. What must occur if a patient refuses to sign the NPP form? _____

    _____

    _____

    _____

    _____

8. How should a medical assistant review a new patient brochure with a new patient? _____

    _____

    _____

    _____

    _____

9. During the check-in process, what three things must the medical assistant do for all patients? _____

    _____

    _____

    _____

    _____

10. If the provider is delayed, what should the medical assistants do with the patients who are waiting?

    _____

    _____

    _____

    _____

11. How should a medical assistant handle a situation when a patient is angry? _____

    _____

    _____

    _____

    _____

12. What occurs during the checkout process? _____

    _____

    _____

    _____

    _____

CERTIFICATION PREPARATION

Cirle the correct answer.

1. The medical assistant may help an angry caller to calm down by
    a. getting angry in return.
    b. speaking in a lower tone of voice.
    c. referring the situation to the office manager immediately.
    d. calling the provider into the situation.

2. Why is it necessary to include a note in the patient's chart when the person does not show up for a scheduled appointment?
    a. To bill the patient for the time
    b. To keep count of the number of no-shows for a possible drop in the future
    c. To be prepared for future legal consequences regarding the patient's care
    d. To provide the medical assistant with a reminder to call and reschedule

3. What is the appointment-setting method by which a patient logs onto the internet and views a facility's schedule to set his or her own appointment?
    a. Flexible office hours
    b. Self-scheduling
    c. Grouping procedures
    d. Advance booking

4. An obstetrician who devotes two afternoons a week to seeing pregnant patients is using an appointment scheduling method called
    a. wave scheduling.
    b. advance booking.
    c. grouping procedures.
    d. modified wave scheduling.

5. Which type of scheduling is an attempt to create short-term flexibility within each hour?
    a. Time-specified scheduling
    b. Wave scheduling
    c. Stream scheduling
    d. Modified-wave scheduling

6. All patients want to be kept informed about how long they should expect to wait to see the provider. Any delay longer than _____ minutes should be explained.
    a. 15
    b. 20
    c. 30
    d. No explanation is necessary

7. When screening patients at the reception desk, which patient has an emergent condition and requires immediate care?
    a. Chest pain
    b. Sore throat
    c. Tick bite
    d. Ankle injury

8. When calling a patient from the reception room to escort him to an exam room, how should the medical assistant call the patient?
    a. "James Brown, Dr. Walden is ready for you."
    b. "James Brown with the sore throat"
    c. "James Brown with a birthdate of June 6"
    d. "James Brown"

9. The statistical characteristics of human populations are called
    a. numbers.
    b. perceptions.
    c. demographics.
    d. phonetics.

10. An effective way to deal with patients who are always late for appointments is to
    a. refuse to schedule them after this happens several times.
    b. have them wait until it is convenient for the physician.
    c. advise them that they disrupt the office schedule.
    d. give them the last appointment of the day.

WORKPLACE APPLICATIONS

1. Janie Haynes consistently arrives at the clinic between 15 and 45 minutes late. She always has a "good" excuse, but she could make her appointments on time if she had better time management skills. The office manager has mentioned to Paula, the receptionist, that Janie is to be scheduled at 4:45 PM and if she is late, she will not be seen by the provider. Paula books Janie's next three appointments at that time, and Janie actually arrives early. However, on the fourth appointment, Janie arrives at 5:50 PM, and Paula knows that it is her responsibility to tell Janie that she cannot see the provider. How does Paula handle this task? What are the options for Paula?

    _____

    _____

    _____

    _____

    _____

2. Jill is the receptionist for Drs. Boles and Bailey, who are psychiatrists. Each week, Sara Ables comes to her appointments but brings her two small children, Joey and Julie, ages 8 and 6 years, respectively. When Sara goes back for her appointment, the children are almost uncontrollable in the reception area. Although there are never more than two patients waiting, the kids are a serious disruption in the clinic. When Jill mentioned the problem to Dr. Boles, he said that Sara really needed the sessions and that Jill should try to work with Sara on this issue. What can Jill do to remedy the situation?

    _____

    _____

    _____

    _____

    _____

INTERNET ACTIVITIES

1. Using online resources, research group appointments. Create a poster presentation, a PowerPoint presentation, or write a paper summarizing your research. Include the following points in your project:
    a. Description of a group appointment
    b. List the types of conditions that are best suited for group appointments
    c. Explain whose confidentiality is maintained with group appointments
    d. List the benefits for patients and providers when group appointments are used

Procedure 11.1   Establish the Appointment Matrix

Name _____ Date _____ Score _____

Task: To establish the matrix of the appointment schedule.

Scenario: You have been asked to set up the schedule matrix for Dr. Julie Walden, Dr. James Martin, and Dr. Angela Perez. Block off the following times in the appointment schedule:

Dr. Julie Walden:
- Lunch; daily from 11:30 AM to 12:30 PM
- Hospital Rounds; Mondays and Wednesday from 8:00 AM to 9:00 AM

Dr. James Martin:
- Lunch; daily from 12:00 PM to 1:00 PM
- Hospital Rounds; Tuesdays and Thursday from 8:00 AM to 9:00 AM

Dr. Angela Perez:
- Lunch; daily from 12:30 PM to 1:30 PM
- Hospital Rounds; Fridays from 8:00 AM to 9:00 AM

Equipment and Supplies:
- Appointment book or computer with scheduling software
- Office procedure manual (optional)
- Black pen, pencil, and highlighters
- Calendar

Standard: Complete the procedure and all critical steps in _____ minutes with a minimum score of 85% within two attempts (*or as indicated by the instructor*).

Scoring: Divide the points earned by the total possible points. Failure to perform a critical step, indicated by an asterisk (*), results in grade no higher than an 84% (*or as indicated by the instructor*).

Time: Began_____ Ended_____ Total minutes: _____

Steps:	Point Value	Attempt 1	Attempt 2
1. Using the calendar, determine when the office is not open (e.g., holidays, weekends, evenings). If using the appointment book and a black pen, draw an *X* through the times the office is not open. If using the scheduling software, block the times the office is not open.	25*		
2. Identify the times each provider is not available. If using the appointment book, write in the providers' names on each column and then draw an *X* through their unavailable times. If using the scheduling software, select each provider and block the times the provider is unavailable.	25*		
3. Using the office procedure manual or providers' preferences, determine when each provider performs certain types of examinations. In the appointment book, indicate these examinations either by writing the examination time or by highlighting the examination times. Follow the office's procedure on indicating these examination times in the appointment book. When using scheduling software, set up the times for the examinations or use the highlighting feature if available.	25*		

4.	Using the office procedure manual or the list of providers' preferences and availability, identify other times to block on the scheduling matrix. Some providers require catch-up times and these time slots are blocked. Some medical facilities save appointment times for same-day appointments. When saving time blocks for same-day appointments, make sure to use pencil so it can be erased and the patient's information entered on the day of the appointment. For the scheduling software, block those times when patients cannot be booked and indicate the times for the same-day appointments.	25*		
	Total Points	100		

Comments

CAAHEP Competencies	Steps
VI.P.1. Manage appointment schedule using established priorities	Entire procedure
ABHES Competencies	**Steps**
7. Administrative Procedures e. Apply scheduling principles	Entire procedure

Procedure 11.2   Schedule a New Patient

Name _____ Date _____ Score _____

Task: To schedule a new patient for a first office visit and identify the urgency of the visit using established priorities.

Scenario: Patricia Black, a new patient, calls. She just moved to the area and her asthma has flared up over the last 24 hours, but her albuterol inhaler is empty, and she needs a new prescription for it. She states that she is doing okay, but without the albuterol she knows it will get worse within the next few days. According to your screening guidelines, she needs to be seen today and scheduling guidelines indicate she needs a 45-minute appointment.

Equipment and Supplies:
- Appointment book or computer with scheduling software
- Scheduling and screening guidelines
- Pencil

Standard: Complete the procedure and all critical steps in _____ minutes with a minimum score of 85% within two attempts (*or as indicated by the instructor*).

Scoring: Divide the points earned by the total possible points. Failure to perform a critical step, indicated by an asterisk (*), results in grade no higher than an 84% (*or as indicated by the instructor*).

Time: Began_____ Ended_____ Total minutes: _____

Steps:	Point Value	Attempt 1	Attempt 2
1. Obtain the patient's demographic information (e.g., full name, birth date, address, and telephone number). Write this information down or enter it into the scheduling software. Verify the information.	15*		
2. Determine whether the patient was referred by another provider.	10		
3. Determine the patient's chief complaint and when the first symptoms occurred. Utilize the scheduling and screening guidelines as needed. *(Refer to the Checklist for Affective Behaviors)*	15*		
4. Search the appointment book or scheduling software for the first suitable appointment time and an alternate time. Offer the patient a choice of these dates and times. Be open to alternative times if the patient cannot make the initial options you gave. Provide additional appointment options as needed.	10*		
5. Enter the mutually agreeable time into the schedule. Enter the patient's name, telephone number, and add *NP* for new patient.	10		
6. Obtain the patient's insurance information. If new patients are expected to pay at the time of the visit, explain this financial arrangement when the appointment is made.	15*		
7. Provide the patient with directions to the healthcare facility and parking instructions if needed.	10		
8. Before ending the call, ask if the patient has any questions. Reinforce the date and time of the appointment. Politely and professionally end the call, making sure to thank the patient for calling. *(Refer to the Checklist for Affective Behaviors)*	15		
Total Points	100		

Checklist for Affective Behaviors

Affective Behavior	*Directions:* Check behaviors observed during the role-play.					
Respect	**Negative, Unprofessional Behaviors**	**Attempt**		**Positive, Professional Behaviors**	**Attempt**	
		1	**2**		**1**	**2**
	Rude, unkind			Courteous		
	Disrespectful, impolite			Polite		
	Unwelcoming			Welcoming		
	Brief, abrupt			Took time with patient		
	Unconcerned with person's dignity			Maintained person's dignity		
	Negative nonverbal behaviors			Positive nonverbal behaviors		
	Other:			Other:		
Sensitivity	Distracted; not focused on the other person			Focused full attention on the other person		
	Judgmental attitude; not accepting attitude			Nonjudgmental, accepting attitude		
	Failed to clarify what the person verbally or nonverbally communicated			Used summarizing or paraphrasing to clarify what the person verbally or nonverbally communicated		
	Failed to acknowledge what the person communicated			Acknowledged what the person communicated		
	Rude, discourteous			Pleasant and courteous		
	Disregarded the person's dignity and rights			Maintained the person's dignity and rights		
	Other:			Other:		

Grading for Affective Behaviors		Point Value	Attempt 1	Attempt 2
Does not meet Expectation	• Response was disrespectful and/or insensitive. • Student demonstrated more than 2 negative, unprofessional behaviors during the interaction.	0		
Needs Improvement	• Response was disrespectful and/or insensitive. • Student demonstrated 1 or 2 negative, unprofessional behaviors during the interaction.	0		
Meets Expectation	• Response was respectful and sensitive; no negative, unprofessional behaviors observed. • More practice is needed for behavior to appear natural and for student to appear comfortable and at ease.	15		
Occasionally Exceeds Expectation	• Response was respectful and sensitive; no negative, unprofessional behaviors observed. • At times student appeared comfortable and at ease; but more practice is needed for behavior to become natural and consistent with a professional medical assistant.	15		
Always Exceeds Expectation	• Response was respectful and sensitive; no negative, unprofessional behaviors observed. • Student's behaviors appeared natural and comfortable. Behaviors are consistent with a professional medical assistant.	15		

Comments

CAAHEP Competencies	Step(s)
VI.P.1. Manage appointment schedule using established priorities	1-7
VI.A.1. Display sensitivity when managing appointments	3, 8
VII.P.3. Obtain accurate patient billing information	6
ABHES Competencies	**Step(s)**
7. Administrative Procedures e. Apply scheduling principles	1-7

Procedure 11.3   Coach Patients Regarding Office Policies

Name _____ **Date** _____ **Score** _____

Tasks: Create a new patient brochure and then role-play ways to coach patients regarding office policies.

Scenario: You work at Walden-Martin Family Medical Clinic. Your supervisor asks you to create a new patient brochure for the clinic. The healthcare facility's information is listed here. After you complete the brochure, you coach the following patients regarding office procedures:
- Mr. Charles Johnson (he has a question regarding the payment policy)
- Ms. Monique Jones (she has a question regarding the medication refill procedure)

Healthcare Facility	Providers
Walden-Martin Family Medical Clinic 1234 Anystreet Anytown, Anystate 12345 Phone: 123-123-1234 Fax: 123-123-5678	Julie Walden, M.D. James Martin, M.D. Angela Perez, M.D. David Kahn, M.D. Jean Burke, N.P.

Equipment and Supplies:
- Computer with word processing software and printer
- Office procedure manual (optional)

Standard: Complete the procedure and all critical steps with a minimum score of 85% within two attempts (*or as indicated by the instructor*).

Scoring: Divide the points earned by the total possible points. Failure to perform a critical step, indicated by an asterisk (*), results in grade no higher than an 84% (*or as indicated by the instructor*).

Steps:	Point Value	Attempt 1	Attempt 2

1. Using word processing software, design an informational brochure for patients that provides information about the healthcare facility and describes practice procedures. At a minimum, the information should include the following:
  a. Description of the healthcare facility (e.g., type of practice, mission statement)
  b. Location or a map of the facility
  c. Contact information (i.e., telephone numbers, emails, and website addresses)
  d. Providers' names and credentials
  e. Services offered
  f. Hours of operation
  g. How appointments can be scheduled
  h. Healthcare facility's policies and procedures (e.g., payment policies, appointment cancellations, medication refills, assistance after hours)
  i. Insurance plans accepted
	55		

2. Proofread the brochure. Revise as needed. Print the brochure.	5		
3. Using the scenario for the first patient, give a brief summary of the different parts of the brochure. Use words the patient will understand.	10*		

4.	Ask if the patient has any questions. Actively listen to the patient's concerns. Address those concerns.	**10***		
5.	Using the scenario for the second patient, give a brief summary of the different parts of the brochure. Use words that the patient understands.	**10***		
6.	Ask if the patient has any questions. Actively listen to the patient's concerns. Address those concerns.	**10***		
	Total Points	**100**		

Comments

CAAHEP Competencies	Step(s)
V.P.4.a. Coach patients regarding: office policies	3-6

Procedure 11.4 Schedule an Established Patient

Name _____ Date _____ Score _____

Task: To manage the provider's schedule by scheduling appointments for an established patient and handling rescheduling and a no-show appointment.

Scenario: Celia Tapia has just finished seeing Dr. Martin and is checking out at your desk. You see that she needs to schedule a follow-up appointment in 2 weeks. The scheduling guidelines indicate a follow-up appointment is 15 minutes long.

Equipment and Supplies:
- Appointment book or computer with scheduling software
- Scheduling guidelines
- Pencil, red pen
- Reminder card
- Patient's health record

Standard: Complete the procedure and all critical steps in _____ minutes with a minimum score of 85% within two attempts (*or as indicated by the instructor*).

Scoring: Divide the points earned by the total possible points. Failure to perform a critical step, indicated by an asterisk (*), results in grade no higher than an 84% (*or as indicated by the instructor*).

Time: Began_____ Ended_____ Total minutes: _____

Steps:	Point Value	Attempt 1	Attempt 2
1. Obtain the patient's name and information, purpose of the visit, the provider to be seen, and any scheduling preferences. If using the scheduling software, enter the patient's name and date of birth (DOB). Verify the correct patient is selected.	15		
2. Identify the length of the appointment by using the scheduling guidelines.	15*		
3. Search the appointment book or scheduling software for the first suitable appointment time and an alternate time. Offer the patient a choice of these dates and times. Be open to alternative times if the patient cannot make the initial options you gave. Provide additional appointment options as needed.	15		
4. Using a pencil, write the patient's name and phone number in the appointment book and block out the correct amount of time. Add in any other relevant information per the facility's procedures. If using the scheduling software, create the appointment per the facility's guidelines.	15*		
5. Complete the appointment reminder card and ensure the date and time on the card matches the appointment time. Give the card to the patient.	10		

Procedure 11.5   Schedule a Patient Procedure

Name _____ Date _____ Score _____

Task: To schedule a patient for a procedure within the time frame needed by the provider, confirm with the patient, and issue all required instructions.

Scenario: Monique Jones has just completed seeing Dr. Walden and is checking out at your desk. She gives you an order from the provider that states she needs to have a magnetic resonance image (MRI) of her left ankle within a week. The radiology department in your facility performs MRIs.

Equipment and Supplies:
- Provider's order detailing the procedure required
- Computer with order entry software (optional)
- Name, address, and telephone number of facility where procedure will take place
- Patient's demographic and insurance information
- Patient's health record
- Procedure preparation instructions
- Telephone
- Consent form (if required for procedure)

Standard: Complete the procedure and all critical steps in _____ minutes with a minimum score of 85% within two attempts (*or as indicated by the instructor*).

Scoring: Divide the points earned by the total possible points. Failure to perform a critical step, indicated by an asterisk (*), results in grade no higher than an 84% (*or as indicated by the instructor*).

Time: Began_____ Ended_____ Total minutes: _____

Steps:	Point Value	Attempt 1	Attempt 2
1. Obtain an oral or written order from the provider for the exact procedure to be performed.	15		
2. Gather the patient's demographic and insurance information. If using an electronic health record, verify you have the correct patient. (*Refer to the Checklist for Affective Behaviors*)	15		
3. Determine the patient's availability within the time frame provided by the provider for the procedure.	15		
4. Contact the diagnostic facility and schedule the patient's procedure. If you are using a computerized provider order entry (CPOE) system and your facility performs the procedure, you also need to enter the order using the CPOE system. • Provide the patient's diagnosis and provider's exact order, including the name of procedure and time frame. • Establish the date and time for the procedure. • Give the patient's name, age, address, telephone number, and insurance information (i.e., insurance policy numbers, precertification information, and addresses for filing claims). • Determine any special instructions for the patient or special anesthesia requirements. • Notify the facility of any urgency for test results.	20*		

5.	If a consent form is required for the procedure, ensure the provider has reviewed the form with the patient and the patient has signed the consent form. A copy of the consent form may be required by the diagnostic facility before the procedure. The consent form should be scanned and uploaded into the electronic health record or placed in the paper record.	15		
6.	Document the details of the scheduled procedure in the patient's health record. If applicable, create a reminder to check on the procedure results after the appointment date.	20*		
	Total Points	100		

Checklist for Affective Behaviors

Affective Behavior	*Directions:* Check behaviors observed during the role-play.					
Respectful	**Negative, Unprofessional Behaviors**	**Attempt**		**Positive, Professional Behaviors**	**Attempt**	
		1	2		1	2
	Rude, unkind			Courteous		
	Disrespectful, impolite			Polite		
	Unwelcoming			Welcoming		
	Brief, abrupt			Took time with patient		
	Unconcerned with person's dignity			Maintained person's dignity		
	Negative nonverbal behaviors			Positive nonverbal behaviors		
	Other:			Other:		
Sensitivity	Distracted; not focused on the other person			Focused full attention on the other person		
	Judgmental attitude; not accepting attitude			Nonjudgmental, accepting attitude		
	Failed to clarify what the person verbally or nonverbally communicated			Used summarizing or paraphrasing to clarify what the person verbally or nonverbally communicated		
	Failed to acknowledge what the person communicated			Acknowledged what the person communicated		
	Rude, discourteous			Pleasant and courteous		
	Disregarded the person's dignity and rights			Maintained the person's dignity and rights		
	Other:			Other:		

Grading for Affective Behaviors		Point Value	Attempt 1	Attempt 2
Does not meet Expectation	• Response was disrespectful and/or insensitive. • Student demonstrated more than 2 negative, unprofessional behaviors during the interaction.	0		
Needs Improvement	• Response was disrespectful and/or insensitive. • Student demonstrated 1 or 2 negative, unprofessional behaviors during the interaction.	0		
Meets Expectation	• Response was respectful and sensitive; no negative, unprofessional behaviors observed. • More practice is needed for behavior to appear natural and for student to appear comfortable and at ease.	15		
Occasionally Exceeds Expectation	• Response was respectful and sensitive; no negative, unprofessional behaviors observed. • At times student appeared comfortable and at ease; but more practice is needed for behavior to become natural and consistent with a professional medical assistant.	15		
Always Exceeds Expectation	• Response was respectful and sensitive; no negative, unprofessional behaviors observed. • Student's behaviors appeared natural and comfortable. Behaviors are consistent with a professional medical assistant.	15		

Comments

CAAHEP Competencies	Steps
VI.P.2. Schedule a patient procedure	All
VI.A.1. Display sensitivity when managing appointments	2
ABHES Competencies	**Steps**
7. Administrative Procedures e. Apply scheduling principles	All

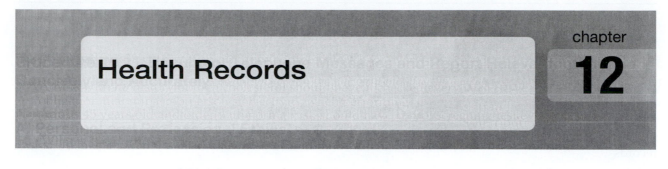

Health Records

CAAHEP Competencies	Assessment
VI.C.4. Define types of information contained in the patient's medical record	Vocabulary Review – A. 1, 7 Skills and Concepts – A. 1, 4
VI.C.5.a. Identify methods of organizing the patient's medical record based on: problem-oriented medical record (POMR)	Skills and Concepts – B. 1
VI.C.5.b. Identify methods of organizing the patient's medical record based on: source-oriented medical record (SOMR)	Vocabulary Review – C. 5, 9, 10 Skills and Concepts – B. 2
VI.C.6.a. Identify equipment and supplies needed for medical records in order to: Create	Skills and Concepts – B. 3
VI.C.6.b. Identify equipment and supplies needed for medical records in order to: Maintain	Skills and Concepts – B. 3
VI.C.6.c. Identify equipment and supplies needed for medical records in order to: Store	Skills and Concepts – B. 3
VI.C.7. Describe filing indexing rules	Skills and Concepts – C. 1
VI.C.11. Explain the importance of data back-up	Skills and Concepts – A. 2
VI.C.12. Explain meaningful use as it applies to EMR	Skills and Concepts – A. 3; Workplace Applications – 1; Internet Activities – 1
VI.P.3. Create a patient's medical record	Procedure 12.1, 12.4
VI.P.4. Organize a patient's medical record	Procedure 12.2, 12.4
VI.P.5. File patient medical records	Procedure 12.2, 12.4, 12.5
VI.P.6. Utilize an EMR	Procedure 12.2
VI.P.7. Input patient data utilizing a practice management system	Procedure 12.1, 12.2
X.A.2. Protect the integrity of the medical record	Procedure 12.1, 12.2, 12.3
ABHES Competencies	**Assessment**
1. General Orientation d. List the general responsibilities and skills of the medical assistant	Skills and Concepts – B.4
4. Medical Law and Ethics a. Follow documentation guidelines	Skills and Concepts – B. 5-9

ABHES Competencies	Assessment
4. Medical Law and Ethics b. Institute federal and state guidelines when: 1) Releasing medical records or information 2) Entering orders in and utilizing electronic health records	Procedure 12.1, 12.2
7. Administrative Procedures a. Gather and process documents	Procedure 12.2, 12.4, 12.5
7. Administrative Procedures b. Navigate electronic health records systems and practice management software	Procedure 12.1, 12.2

VOCABULARY REVIEW

Using the word pool on the right, find the correct word to match the definition. Write the word on the line after the definition.

Group A

1. Data or information obtained from the patient
   _____

2. A process to ensure the reliability of test results
   _____

3. Using as few words as possible to express the message
   _____

4. A computerized record that conforms to nationally recognized standards and contains health-related information about a specific patient _____

5. A temporary diagnosis made before all test results have been received _____

6. The smooth continuation of care from one provider to another that allows the patient to receive the most benefit and no interruption or duplication of care _____

7. Data obtained through physical examination, laboratory and diagnostic testing, and by measurable information
   _____

8. The likely outcome of a disease including chance of recovery
   _____

9. Passed from parents to offspring through the genes
   _____

10. How often something happens _____

Word Pool
- electronic health record (EHR)
- quality control
- prognosis
- continuity of care
- incidence
- subjective information
- objective information
- hereditary
- concise
- provisional diagnosis

Group B

1. The ability to work with other systems _____

2. A method or plan for retaining or keeping health records and for their movement from active to inactive to closed _____

3. Occurring later or after _____

4. A rule that controls how something should be done; guidelines or boundaries _____

5. An interconnection between systems _____

6. A secure online website that gives patients 24-hour access to personal health information using a username and password _____

7. The use of electronic software to communicate with pharmacies and send prescribing information _____

8. The process of entering medication orders or other provider instructions into the EHR _____

9. Meeting the standards and regulations of the practice's established policies and procedures _____

10. Granted or endowed with a particular authority, right, or property; to have a special interest in _____

Word Pool
- subsequent
- patient portal
- vested
- interoperability
- e-prescribing
- compliance
- computerized provider/physician order entry (CPOE)
- parameters
- interface
- retention schedule

Group C

1. The age at which a person is recognized by law to be an adult; it varies by state _____

2. A heading, title, or subtitle under which records are filed _____

3. To say something aloud for another person to write down _____

4. A chronologic file used as a reminder that something must be dealt with on a certain date _____

5. The filing of records, correspondence, or cards by number _____

6. To make a written copy of dictated material _____

7. A sturdy cardboard or plastic file-sized card used to replace a folder temporarily removed from the filing space _____

8. To remove or destroy all traces of; do away with; destroy completely _____

9. The most recent item is on top and oldest item is last _____

10. Any system that arranges names or topics according to the sequence of the letters in the alphabet _____

Word Pool
- age of majority
- reverse chronologic order
- obliteration
- transcription
- dictation
- out guides
- caption
- alphabetic filing
- numeric filing
- tickler file

ABBREVIATIONS
Write out what each of the following abbreviations stands for.

1. AMA _____

2. CPOE _____

3. CPT _____

4. EHRs _____

5. HHS _____

6. HIE _____

7. HIPAA _____

8. HIV _____

9. ICD _____

10. NPP _____

11. ONC _____

12. PCP _____

13. PHI _____

14. PHR _____

15. POR _____

16. SOR _____

17. TPR _____

SKILLS AND CONCEPTS
Answer the following questions. Write your answer on the line or in the space provided.

A. Health Record Basics

1. Describe the following types of information found in a patient's health record.

    Demographics: _____

    _____

    _____

    _____

    _____

    _____

Past health history: _____

_____

_____

_____

_____

_____

_____

Family history:_____

_____

_____

_____

_____

_____

_____

Social history: _____

_____

_____

_____

_____

_____

_____

Chief complaint: _____

_____

_____

_____

_____

_____

_____

4. Describe the medical assistant's responsibilities when documenting in the health record including skills and responsibilities.

_____

_____

_____

_____

_____

_____

_____

Correct the following entries as would be done in the health record. Then rewrite the entries correctly. Handwritten corrections are acceptable on these exercises.

5. The correct date of the appointment below was October 12, 20XX.

   10-21-20XX 1330 Patient did not arrive for scheduled appointment. P. Smith, RMA

   _____

   _____

   _____

   _____

6. The patient stated that the chest pain began 2 weeks ago.

   1-31-20XX 10:00 AM Patient complained of chest pain for the past 2 months. No pain noted in arms. No nausea. Desires ECG and blood work to check for heart problems. R. Smithee, CMA (AAMA)

   _____

   _____

   _____

   _____

Document the following exercises.

7. Eric Robertson canceled his surgical follow-up appointment today for the third time. Document this information.

   _____

   _____

   _____

   _____

8. Angela Adams called to report that she was not feeling any better since her office visit on Monday. She wants the doctor to call in a refill for her antibiotics. The chart says that she was to return to the clinic on Thursday if she was not feeling better. Today is Monday, and she says she cannot come into the clinic this week. The physician wants to see her before prescribing any other medication. Document this information.

_____

_____

_____

_____

_____

_____

9. Mary Elizabeth Smith called the physician's office to report redness around an injection site. She was in the office 3 hours ago and received an injection of penicillin. She says she also is itching quite a bit around the site and is having trouble breathing. The doctor has left the office for the day. Office policy states that if the physician is out of the office and a patient presents or calls with an emergency, he or she is to be referred to the ER. Document the action that the medical assistant should take.

_____

_____

_____

_____

_____

_____

C. Indexing and Filing Rules

1. Describe the indexing rules for alphabetic filing. _____

_____

_____

_____

_____

_____

_____

_____

_____

2. Using alphabetic filing, place the names below in correct alphabetic order.

Cassidy Kay Hale	1. _____
Candace Cassidy LeGrand	2. _____
Taylor Ann Jackson	3. _____
Anton Douglas Conn	4. _____
Mitchel Michael Gibson	5. _____
Lorienda Gaye Robison	6. _____
LaNelle Elva Crumley	7. _____
Allison Gaile Yarbrough	8. _____
Sarah Kay Haile	9. _____
Marie Gracelia Stuart	10. _____
Karry Madge Chapmann	11. _____
Randi Ann Perez	12. _____
Cecelia Gayle Raglan	13. _____
Sarah Sue Ragland	14. _____
Riley Americus Belk	15. _____
Starr Ellen Beall	16. _____
Mitchell Thomas Gibson	17. _____
George Scott Turner	18. _____
Winston Roger Murchison	19. _____
Sara Suzelle Montgomery	20. _____
Tamika Noelle Frazier	21. _____
Alisa Jordan Williams	22. _____
Alisha Dawn Chapman	23. _____
Bentley James Adams	24. _____
Montana Skye Kizer	25. _____
Dakota Marie LaRose	26. _____
Robbie Sue Metzger	27. _____
Thomas Charles Bruin	28. _____
Percival "Butch" Adams	29. _____
Carlos Perez Santos	30. _____

3. Why might color-coded files be more efficient than an alphabetic filing system? _____

_____

_____

_____

_____

_____

_____

4. Using terminal filing, place the numbers below in the correct order.

01-64-22	1. _____
72-55-20	2. _____
44-41-20	3. _____
17-41-20	4. _____
56-42-21	5. _____
91-88-21	6. _____
15-24-22	7. _____
82-49-20	8. _____
08-94-21	9. _____
24-42-22	10. _____

D. Miscellaneous

1. Describe the difference between an EMR and a practice management system. _____

_____

_____

_____

_____

_____

2. Describe a manual tickler file. _____

_____

_____

_____

_____

3. Correspondence related to the operation of the of the office is considered _____ correspondence.

CERTIFICATION PREPARATION

Circle the correct answer.

1. Information that is obtained by questioning the patient or that is taken from a form is called _____ information.
   a. confidential
   b. subjective
   c. necessary
   d. objective

2. How would you properly index the name "Amanda M. Stiles-Duncan" for filing?
   a. Stilesduncan, Amanda M.
   b. Stiles Duncan, Amanda M.
   c. Duncanstiles, Amanda M.
   d. Duncan, Amanda M. Stiles

3. Who is the legal owner of the information stored in a patient's record?
   a. The patient
   b. The provider or agency where services were provided
   c. The patient's insurance company
   d. Both the patient and the provider

4. Which is *not* objective information?
   a. Progress notes
   b. Family history
   c. Diagnosis
   d. Physical examination and findings

5. Many healthcare facilities now use voice recognition software for transcription. The system can be used to dictate which types of reports?
   a. Progress notes
   b. Letters
   c. Emails
   d. All of the above

6. Perhaps the most essential action for the medical assistant working with a patient and using an electronic record is to
   a. type in every word the patient says.
   b. make sure the patient is not hiding any part of the health history.
   c. make frequent eye contact with patient and smile.
   d. sit in a chair across from the patient so that the person cannot see the screen.

7. Which EHR system backup requires the least amount of hardware?
   a. Online backup system
   b. External hard drives
   c. Full server backup
   d. Thumb drive backup

8. The concise account of the patient's symptoms in his or her own words is the _____.
   a. Objective information
   b. Provisional diagnosis
   c. Chief complaint
   d. Caption

9. To completely remove all traces of an entry in a health record is _____.
   a. interface
   b. obliteration
   c. dictation
   d. compliance

10. The process of electronic data entry of a provider's instructions for the treatment of patients is called _____.
    a. progress notes
    b. computerized physician/provider order entry
    c. direct filing system
    d. continuity of care

WORKPLACE APPLICATIONS

1. Dr. Martin wants to be sure the Walden-Martin Family Medical (WMFM) Clinic is meeting all of the requirements for meaningful use that are specified in the HITECH Act. He has asked Susan to put together a list of what WMFM Clinic should be doing to meet those requirements. What would be on Susan's list?

    _____

    _____

    _____

    _____

2. Susan has been learning about the various EHR systems available. She has also been learning about the need to back up to protect the information stored in the EHR. Susan has asked the office manager at WMFC how the EHR is backed up at their facility. The office manager states that they currently use an external hard drive, but would like to look more closely at other options. She asks Susan to determine what other options are available. Write a brief description of each of the options below:

    a. External hard drive:_____

    _____

    b. Full server backup: _____

    _____

    c. Online backup system: _____

    _____

INTERNET ACTIVITIES

1. Using online resources, research EHR systems. Choose the one you think would be the best option and create a poster presentation, a PowerPoint presentation, or write a paper summarizing your research. Include the following points in your project:
    a. Description of the EHR
    b. Description of the practice management functions
    c. Does it include backup features?
    d. How does it meet the meaningful use requirements?

2. Using online resources, research a voice recognition software. Create a poster presentation, a PowerPoint presentation, or write a paper summarizing your research. Include the following points in your project:
    a. Description voice recognition software
    b. List the uses for voice recognition software
    c. Compare three different products
    d. Determine which one would be the best product

Checklist for Affective Behaviors

Affective Behavior	Directions: *Check behaviors observed during the role-play.*					
Ethical	Failed to adequately follow the facility's policy			Adequately followed the facility's policy		
	Incorrectly entered patient's information (e.g., misspelled name) during the database search			Correctly entered patient's information (e.g., misspelled name) when searching database		
	Incorrectly entered patient's information (e.g., misspelled name) when registering patient			Correctly entered patient's information (e.g., misspelled name) when registering patient		
	Other:			Other:		

Grading for Affective Behaviors		Point Value	Attempt 1	Attempt 2
Does not meet Expectation	• Response was unethical. • Student demonstrated more than 2 negative, unprofessional behaviors during the interaction.	0		
Needs Improvement	• Response was unethical • Student demonstrated 1 or 2 negative, unprofessional behaviors during the interaction.	0		
Meets Expectation	• Response was ethical; no negative, unprofessional behaviors observed. • More practice is needed for behavior to appear natural and for student to appear comfortable and at ease.	15		
Occasionally Exceeds Expectation	• Response was ethical; no negative, unprofessional behaviors observed. • At times student appeared comfortable and at ease; but more practice is needed for behavior to become natural and consistent with a professional medical assistant.	15		
Always Exceeds Expectation	• Response was ethical; no negative, unprofessional behaviors observed. • Student's behaviors appeared natural and comfortable. Behaviors are consistent with a professional medical assistant.	15		

CAAHEP Competencies	Steps
VI.P.3. Create a patient's medical record	All
X.A.2. Protect the integrity of the medical record	2, 4
ABHES Competencies	**Steps**
7. Administrative Procedures b. Navigate electronic health records systems and practice management software	All

Figure 12.1   Patient Information Form

Patient Information:
Name: Jonathan S. Scott
Address: 922 Golf Road, Anytown, AK 12345
Date of Birth: 08/01/1990
Email: jscott16@anytown.mail
Sex: M
Home Phone: 123-123-3098
SSN: 987-66-1223
Emergency Contact Name: Callie Scott
Emergency Contact Phone: 123-123-0857

Guarantor Information:
Relationship of Guarantor to Patient: Self
Employer Name: Anytown Bank
Work Phone: 123-567-9012
Primary Provider: David Kahn, MD

Insurance Information:
   Primary Insurance:
       Insurance: Aetna
       Name of Policyholder: Jonathan S. Scott
       SSN of Policyholder: 987-66-1223
       Policy/ID Number: JS8884910
       Group Number: 66574W
       Claims Address: 1234 Insurance Way, Anytown, AL 12345-1234
       Claims Phone Number: 180-012-3222

Procedure 12.2   Upload Documents to the EHR

Name _____ Date _____ Score _____

Task: Scan paper records and upload digital files to the EHR.

Scenario: A new patient brings in a laboratory report and a radiology report that he would like to have added to his EHR. You need to scan in the original documents and upload them to the EHR.

Equipment and Supplies:
- Scanner
- Computer with SimChart for the Medical Office or EHR software
- Patient's laboratory and radiology reports (Figures 12.2 and 12.3)

Standard: Complete the procedure and all critical steps in _____ minutes with a minimum score of 85% within two attempts (*or as indicated by the instructor*).

Scoring: Divide the points earned by the total possible points. Failure to perform a critical step, indicated by an asterisk (*), results in grade no higher than an 84% (*or as indicated by the instructor*).

Time: Began_____ Ended_____ Total minutes: _____

Steps:	Point Value	Attempt 1	Attempt 2
1. Obtain the patient's name and date of birth if not on the reports.	10		
2. Using a scanner that is connected to the computer, scan each document, creating an individual digital image for each.	20		
3. Locate the file of the two scanned images in the computer drive. Open the files to ensure the images are clear.	15*		
4. To help ensure the integrity of the practice management and EHR systems, a search for the new patient's name must always be done. In the EHR, search for the patient, using the patient's last and first name. Verify the patient's date of birth. *(Refer to the Checklist for Affective Behaviors)*	15*		
5. Locate the window to upload diagnostic/laboratory results and add a new result. Enter the date of the test. Select the correct type of result. Browse for the image file of the laboratory file and attach it. Save the information.	15*		
6. Select the option to add a new result and repeat the steps to upload the second report.	10*		
7. To help ensure the integrity of the EHR system, verify that the correct documents were uploaded and specific headers (titles) were given to the document. *(Refer to the Checklist for Affective Behaviors)*	15*		
Total Points	100		

Checklist for Affective Behaviors

Affective Behavior	**Directions:** *Check behaviors observed during the role-play.*					
Ethical	Failed to adequately follow the facility's policy			Adequately followed the facility's policy		
	Incorrectly entered patient's information (e.g., misspelled name) during the database search			Correctly entered patient's information (e.g., misspelled name) when searching database		
	Incorrectly uploaded a document			Correctly uploaded the document		
	Incorrectly titled the document uploaded			Correctly titled the document uploaded		
	Other:			Other:		

Grading for Affective Behaviors		Point Value	Attempt 1	Attempt 2
Does not meet Expectation	• Response was unethical • Student demonstrated more than 2 negative, unprofessional behaviors during the interaction.	0		
Needs Improvement	• Response was unethical. • Student demonstrated 1 or 2 negative, unprofessional behaviors during the interaction.	0		
Meets Expectation	• Response was ethical; no negative, unprofessional behaviors observed. • More practice is needed for behavior to appear natural and for student to appear comfortable and at ease.	15		
Occasionally Exceeds Expectation	• Response was ethical; no negative, unprofessional behaviors observed. • At times student appeared comfortable and at ease; but more practice is needed for behavior to become natural and consistent with a professional medical assistant.	15		
Always Exceeds Expectation	• Response was ethical; no negative, unprofessional behaviors observed. • Student's behaviors appeared natural and comfortable. Behaviors are consistent with a professional medical assistant.	15		

CAAHEP Competencies	Steps
VI.P.4. Organize a patient's medical record	2-5
VI.P.5. File patient medical records	2-5
X.A.2. Protect the integrity of the medical record	4, 7
ABHES Competencies	**Steps**
7. Administrative Procedures a. Gather and process documents	2-5
7. Administrative Procedures b. Navigate electronic health records systems and practice management software	All

Figure 12.2 Laboratory Report

AnyTown Laboratory

Date Reported:	04/25/20XX	**Date Received:**	04/25/20XX
Patient Name:	Jonathan S. Scott	**DOB:**	08/01/1990
Ordering Provider:	George St. Cyr, MD		
Date Collected:	04/15/20XX	**Time Collected:**	0830
Test Requested:	Lipid Panel	**Fasting?:**	Yes

Test	Result	Flag	Reference Range
Cholesterol, total	210	High	<200 mg/dL
HDL Cholesterol	26	Low	>40 mg/dL
LDL Cholesterol	142	High	<130 mg/dL
Triglycerides	236	High	<150 mg/dL
Total Cholesterol/HDL ratio	5.8	High	<4.5

Figure 12.3   Radiology Report

AnyTown Radiology

Date:	10/31/20XX		**Time:**	1430
Patient Name:	Jonathan S. Scott		**DOB:**	08/01/1990
Exam Type:	Chest x-ray 2 views		**Ordering Provider:**	George St. Cyr, MD

Final Report:
History: Cough and fever
Report: Frontal and lateral views of the chest
Comparison: None

Findings:
Lungs: The lungs are well inflated and clear. There is no evidence of pneumonia or pulmonary edema.
Pleura: There is no pleural effusion or pneumothorax.
Heart and mediastinum: The cardiomediastinal silhouette is normal.
Impression: Clear lungs without evidence of pneumonia.
Recommendation: None.
Provider: Bones, Seymore MD

Procedure 12.3 Protect the Integrity of the Medical Record

Name _____ Date _____ Score _____

Tasks: Protect the integrity of the medical record.

Scenario: You are mentoring a medical assistant student who is in practicum. You notice the student routinely does not sign out of the electronic health record before leaving the desk. The facility's policy is to sign out or lock the computer before leaving it.

Directions: Role-play the scenario with a peer, who plays the student. You, the medical assistant, must explain to the "student" the facility's policy. Also address the hazards of not protecting the medical record. If the student does not change his/her behavior, you will need to address the situation with the department supervisor.

Standard: Complete the procedure and all critical steps in _____ minutes with a minimum score of 85% within two attempts (*or as indicated by the instructor*).

Scoring: Divide the points earned by the total possible points. Failure to perform a critical step, indicated by an asterisk (*), results in grade no higher than an 84% (*or as indicated by the instructor*).

Time: Began_____ Ended_____ Total minutes: _____

Steps:	Point Value	Attempt 1	Attempt 2
1. Professionally and respectfully discuss the situation with the student. (*Refer to the Checklist for Affective Behaviors – Respect.*)	25		
2. Inform the student about the facility's policy and the hazards of not protecting the electronic health record. (*Refer to the Checklist for Affective Behaviors – Ethics.*)	25		
3. Provide the student with strategies to protect the electronic health record. (*Refer to the Checklist for Affective Behaviors – Ethics.*)	25		
4. Inform the student what will occur if he/she does not protect the electronic record. (*Refer to the Checklist for Affective Behaviors – Respect.*)	25		
Total Points	100		

Procedure 12.4   Create and Organize a Patient's Paper Health Record

Name _____ **Date** _____ **Score** _____

Task: Create a paper health record for a new patient. Organize health record documents in a paper health record.

Equipment and Supplies:
- End tab file folder
- Completed patient registration form (Figure 12.1)
- Divider sheets with different color labels (4)
- Progress note sheet (1)
- Name label
- Color-coding labels (first two letters of last name and first letter of first name)
- Year label
- Allergy label
- Black pen or computer with word processing software to process labels
- Health record documents (i.e., prior records, laboratory reports) (Figures 12.2 and 12.3)
- Hole puncher

Standard: Complete the procedure and all critical steps in _____ minutes with a minimum score of 85% within two attempts (*or as indicated by the instructor*).

Scoring: Divide the points earned by the total possible points. Failure to perform a critical step, indicated by an asterisk (*), results in grade no higher than an 84% (*or as indicated by the instructor*).

Time: Began_____ Ended_____ Total minutes: _____

Steps:	Point Value	Attempt 1	Attempt 2
1. Obtain the patient's first and last name.	5		
2. Neatly write or word process the patient's name on the name label. Left-justify the last name, followed by a comma, the first name, middle initial and a period (e.g., Smith, Mary J.).	10		
3. Adhere the name label to the bottom left side of the record tab. When the record is held by the main fold in your left hand, the writing should be easy to read. (For directional purposes, assume the record main fold is on the left and the tab is at the bottom.)	10		
4. Put the color-coding labels on the bottom right edge of the folder. Start by placing the first letter of the last name at the farthest right edge. Working left, place the second letter of the last name, then the first letter of the first name, and lastly the year label. The year label should be close to the name label.	15*		
5. Place the allergy label on the front of the record. If allergies are known, clearly write the allergy on the label in red ink.	10*		
6. Place the divider labels on the record divider sheets, if they come separately. Ensure the labels on the divider sheets are staggered so they do not overlap. Print the name of the section on the front and back of the label. The print should be easy to read when the record is held by the main fold.	10		

7. Using the prongs on the left-hand side of the record, secure the registration form.	**10**		
8. Using the prongs on the right-hand side of the record, secure the index dividers with a progress note sheet under the progress note tab.	**10**		
Scenario Update: The patient authorized his/her prior provider to send health records to your agency. You need to organize these records within the paper health record.			
9. To help ensure the integrity of the practice management and EHR systems, a search for the new patient's name must always be done. This prevents errors in documentation. Verify the name and the date of birth on the health records and ensure they match the information on the health record. *(Refer to the Checklist for Affective Behaviors)*	**10***		
10. Open the prongs on the right side of the record and carefully remove the record to the point of where the documents need to be inserted. For the documents being inserted, punch holes in the proper location. Insert the papers into the record and then reassemble the remaining part of the record. Continue to do this until all the documents are filed within the health record.	**10**		
Total Points	**100**		

Checklist for Affective Behaviors

Affective Behavior	Directions: Check behaviors observed during the role-play.					
Ethical	Fails to adequately explain facility's policy.			Adequate explains the facility's policy.		
	Fails to adequately discuss the hazards of not protecting the paper health record.			Adequately explains the legal and ethical results of not protecting the paper health record. Addresses the consequences to the clinic, employee, and patient.		
	Fails to adequately explain how to protect the paper health record.			Adequately explains how to protect the paper health record (e.g., close files when done, turn so that the patient name is not visible)		
	Other:			Other:		

Grading for Affective Behaviors		Point Value	Attempt 1	Attempt 2
Does not meet Expectation	• Response was disrespectful. • Student demonstrated more than 2 negative, unprofessional behaviors during the interaction.	0		
Needs Improvement	• Response was disrespectful. • Student demonstrated 1 or 2 negative, unprofessional behaviors during the interaction.	0		
Meets Expectation	• Response was respectful; no negative, unprofessional behaviors observed. • More practice is needed for behavior to appear natural and for student to appear comfortable and at ease.	15		
Occasionally Exceeds Expectation	• Response was respectful; no negative, unprofessional behaviors observed. • At times student appeared comfortable and at ease; but more practice is needed for behavior to become natural and consistent with a professional medical assistant.	15		
Always Exceeds Expectation	• Response was respectful; no negative, unprofessional behaviors observed. • Student's behaviors appeared natural and comfortable. Behaviors are consistent with a professional medical assistant.	15		

CAAHEP Competencies	Steps
VI.P.4. Organize a patient's medical record	6, 7, 8, 10
VI.P.5. File patient medical records	10
X.A.2. Protect the integrity of the medical record	9
ABHES Competencies	**Steps**
7. Administrative Procedures a. Gather and process documents	10

Procedure 12.5   File Patient Health Records

Name _____ Date _____ Score _____

Task: File patient health records using two different filing systems: the alphabetic system and the numeric system.

Scenario: The agency utilizes the alphabetic system. You need to file health records in the correct location.

Equipment and Supplies:
- Paper health records using the alphabetic filing system
- Paper health records using the numeric filing system
- File box(es) or file cabinet

Standard: Complete the procedure and all critical steps in _____ minutes with a minimum score of 85% within two attempts (*or as indicated by the instructor*).

Scoring: Divide the points earned by the total possible points. Failure to perform a critical step, indicated by an asterisk (*), results in grade no higher than an 84% (*or as indicated by the instructor*).

Time: Began_____ Ended_____ Total minutes: _____

Steps:	Point Value	Attempt 1	Attempt 2
1. Using alphabetic guidelines, place the records to be filed in alphabetic order.	20		
2. Using the file box or file cabinet, locate the correct spot for the first file.	10		
3. Place the health record in the correct location. Continue these filing steps until all the health records are filed.	20*		
4. Using numeric guidelines, place the records to be filed in numeric order.	20		
5. Using the file box or file cabinet, locate the correct spot for the first file.	10		
6. Place the health record in the correct location. Continue these filing steps until all the health records are filed.	20*		
Total Points	100		

CAAHEP Competencies	Steps
VI.P.5. File patient medical records	3, 6
ABHES Competencies	**Steps**
7. Administrative Procedures a. Gather and process documents	All

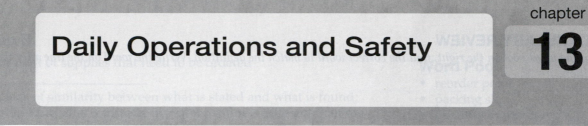

Daily Operations and Safety

chapter

13

CAAHEP Competencies	Assessment
VI.C.9. Explain the purpose of routine maintenance of administrative and clinical equipment	Skills and Concepts – B. 5; Certification Preparation – 5
VI.C.10. List steps involved in completing an inventory	Skills and Concepts – B. 9
VI.P.8. Perform routine maintenance of administrative or clinical equipment	Procedure 13.2
VI.P.9. Perform an inventory with documentation	Procedure 13.1, 13.3
XII.C.3. Discuss fire safety issues in an ambulatory healthcare environment	Skills and Concepts – C. 15-18; Certification Preparation – 7, 9
XII.C.4. Describe fundamental principles for evacuation of a healthcare setting	Skills and Concepts – C. 12-14; Internet Activities – 3
XII.C.7.a. Identify principles of: body mechanics	Skills and Concepts – C. 1-3; Certification Preparation – 6; Workplace Application – 2
XII.C.8. Identify critical elements of an emergency plan for response to a natural disaster or other emergency	Skills and Concepts – C. 8; Certification Preparation – 8; Internet Activities – 3
XII.P.2.b. Demonstrate proper use of: fire extinguishers	Procedure 13.6
XII.P.3. Use proper body mechanics	Procedure 13.4
XII.P.4. Participate in a mock exposure event with documentation of specific steps	Procedure 13.5
XII.P.5. Evaluate the work environment to identify unsafe working conditions	Procedure 13.4
XII.A.1. Recognize the physical and emotional effects on persons involved in an emergency situation	Procedure 13.5
XII.A.2. Demonstrate self-awareness in responding to an emergency situation	Procedure 13.5
ABHES Competencies	**Assessment**
7. Administrative Procedures f. Maintain inventory of equipment and supplies	Procedure 13.1, 13.3

6. Describe three factors that are taken into consideration when deciding to replace a piece of equipment with a newer model.

_____

_____

_____

7. Explain two reasons that a supervisor or provider may opt to lease a piece of equipment versus buying it.

_____

_____

8. List eight items that should be recorded for each supply in inventory. _____

_____

_____

9. List steps involved in completing an inventory. _____

_____

_____

_____

10. Describe the usefulness of purchase order numbers for the vendor and the medical facility. _____

_____

_____

11. On receiving supply deliveries, describe why it is important to check the merchandise as soon as possible.

_____

_____

_____

12. Explain how the packing slip is used when ordered supplies arrive. _____

_____

_____

C. Safety and Security

1. When lifting an object, explain how your feet should be placed. _____

_____

_____

2. Describe the position of your knees and back when lifting. _____

_____

_____

3. List four other principles of body mechanics. _____

_____

_____

_____

4. List four ways to keep safe in the work environment. _____

_____

_____

_____

5. List five high-risk situations inside the facility that can lead to accidents. _____

_____

_____

_____

6. List four ways a medical assistant can help prevent injuries and fires. _____

_____

_____

_____

7. Describe an emergency response plan. _____

_____

_____

_____

8. Identify six critical elements of an emergency plan for response to a natural disaster or other emergency.

_____

_____

_____

9. Floor maps with _____ and _____ should be posted throughout the facility.

10. _____ must be clearly marked and well-lit.

11. Exit routes should be clear of _____ and _____ at all times.

12. List evacuation priorities by locations. Start with the most critical or highest priority to evacuate.

_____

_____

_____

13. List evacuation priorities by people. Start with the most critical or highest priority to evacuate._____

_____

_____

_____

14. Describe the five types of evacuations. _____

_____

_____

_____

_____

_____

15. List five items that should be located throughout the facility per state code for fire response. _____

_____

_____

16. Describe RACE._____

_____

_____

_____

17. Describe PASS or how to use most fire extinguishers. _____

_____

_____

_____

18. What two types of fire extinguishers are used for a paper or wood fire? _____

_____

19. Describe the stages of general adaptation syndrome (GAS)._____

_____

_____

_____

CERTIFICATION PREPARATION

Circle the correct answer.

1. What is an opening task for the administrative medical assistant?
   a. Unlock supply cabinets.
   b. Perform quality-control tests on laboratory equipment.
   c. Update the voicemail message.
   d. Follow up on outstanding patient issues from the prior day.

2. What should be disinfected in the healthcare facility?
   a. Exam table
   b. Writing table
   c. Computer keyboard
   d. All of the above

3. How often do crash carts and other emergency supplies need to be inventoried?
   a. Every week
   b. Every other week
   c. Every month
   d. Every 6 months

4. What is *not* found on a routine maintenance log?
   a. Equipment name, serial number, and location of the machine
   b. Manufacturer's name and date of purchase
   c. Store name where the machine was purchased
   d. Warranty information and service provider information

5. What the purpose of routine maintenance of administrative and clinical equipment?
   a. Prevent injury to the patients
   b. Prevent costly damage to the equipment
   c. Prevent injury to staff members
   d. All of the above

6. What is *not* a principle of proper body mechanics?
   a. When lifting an object, maintain a wide, stable base with your feet.
   b. Get help if the item is too heavy to lift by yourself.
   c. Keep your movements smooth.
   d. When reaching for an object, you can stand on tiptoes.

7. What is the correct way to operate most fire extinguishers?
   a. Pull the pin, squeeze the handle, aim the nozzle, and sweep the nozzle from side to side
   b. Pull the pin, aim the nozzle, sweep the nozzle from side to side, and squeeze the handle
   c. Pull the pin, sweep the nozzle from side to side, squeeze the handle, and aim the nozzle
   d. Pull the pin, aim the nozzle, squeeze the handle, and sweep the nozzle from side to side

8. What is a critical element of an emergency response plan?
   a. Evacuation policy and procedure
   b. Methods to report emergencies
   c. Critical shutdown procedures
   d. All of the above

9. Which is a dry chemical fire extinguisher that is used on fires related to electrical sources?
   a. A
   b. B
   c. C
   d. D

10. Which is *not* a symptom of stress?
    a. Anger
    b. Low blood pressure
    c. Anxiety
    d. Fear

Work Product 13.2 Maintenance Logs

Name _____ Date _____ Score _____

To be used with Procedure 13.2.

Maintenance Log

Equipment: _____ Serial #: _____ Location: _____
Facility #: _____ Manufacturer: _____ Purchased: _____
Warranty Information: _____
Frequency of Inspections: _____
Service Provider: _____

Date	Time	Maintenance Activities	Signature

Maintenance Log

Equipment: _____ Serial #: _____ Location: _____
Facility #: _____ Manufacturer: _____ Purchased: _____
Warranty Information: _____
Frequency of Inspections: _____
Service Provider: _____

Date	Time	Maintenance Activities	Signature

Maintenance Log

Equipment: _____ Serial #: _____ Location: _____
Facility #: _____ Manufacturer: _____ Purchased: _____
Warranty Information: _____
Frequency of Inspections: _____
Service Provider: _____

Date	Time	Maintenance Activities	Signature

Maintenance Log

Equipment: _____ Serial #: _____ Location: _____
Facility #: _____ Manufacturer: _____ Purchased: _____
Warranty Information: _____
Frequency of Inspections: _____
Service Provider: _____

Date	Time	Maintenance Activities	Signature

Procedure 13.3 Perform a Supply Inventory with Documentation While Using Proper Body Mechanics

Name _____ Date _____ Score _____

Tasks: Perform a supply inventory using correct body mechanics. Document the inventory on the supply inventory form.

Equipment and Supplies:
- Pens
- Administrative or clinical supplies to be inventoried
- Purchase information (e.g., item number, cost, and supplier) for supplies in inventory
- Reorder point and quantity to reorder for each item in inventory
- Supply inventory form (Work Product 13.3)

Standard: Complete the procedure and all critical steps with a minimum score of 85% within two attempts (*or as indicated by the instructor*).

Scoring: Divide the points earned by the total possible points. Failure to perform a critical step, indicated by an asterisk (*), results in grade no higher than an 84% (*or as indicated by the instructor*).

Steps:	Point Value	Attempt 1	Attempt 2
1. For the supplies in inventory, gather the following information for each item: • Name, size, quantity (e.g., purchased individually, 100 per box) • Item number, supplier's name, cost • Reorder point and quantity to reorder	5		
2. For each supply item, enter information on the inventory form (Work Product 13.3). Make sure the appropriate entry is in the right location. Note: The "Stock Available" column will be empty for now.	15*		
3. Review the document. Make any necessary revisions.	10		
4. Using the supply inventory list, inventory the supplies in the department. Identify how the supply should be counted (e.g., individually, by the box) and count the number of items in stock.	15		
5. Add the number in the appropriate row under the "Stock Available" header.	10		
6. Compare the reorder point number to the stock available number. If the stock available number is at or below the reorder point, indicate that the item needs to be reordered by checking the appropriate column.	10*		
7. Make sure the supplies are neatly arranged. The older stock should be in front of the newer stock.	5		
8. Repeat steps 5 through 7 until all supplies are inventoried.	10		
9. Use proper body mechanics when lifting and moving supplies by maintaining a wide, stable base with your feet. Your feet should be shoulder-width apart and you should have good footing. Bend at the knees, keeping your back straight. Lift smoothly with the major muscles in your arms and legs. Use the same technique when putting the item down.	10*		

Work Product 13.4   Work Environment Evaluation Form

Name _____   **Date** _____   **Score** _____
To be used with Procedure 13.4.

Directions: *Check either in the "Yes" or "No" column for each question. Check "NA" if it is not applicable. Include any issues in the comment column. Summarize your findings for each area, using the space indicated.*

Slipping, tripping, or fall risks	Yes	No	NA	Comments
• Is the lighting appropriate?				
• Are any lights burned out? Are any areas dim?				
• Is the flooring and carpeting ripped or pulled up?				
• If rugs/mats are present, are they folded?				
• Is water on the floor?				
• Is signage present warning of the water?				
• Are items cluttering the hallway, making walking difficult?				
• Are cords, cables, and other items in the walkway?				
• Is trash on the floor?				
• Are heavy items on high shelves?				
• Is a sturdy step stool available?				
Safety and security issues	Yes	No	NA	Comments
• Are rooms available that can be locked and used during workplace violence?				
• Is there limited visibility from the hallway into the room?				
• Are there areas in the building with limited visibility?				
• If the building is accessible to the public, are there any safe zones or areas for staff?				
• Are the emergency call lights in the exam rooms and bathrooms functioning?				
• Are the oxygen tanks (if available) checked per the facility's policy?				
Fire risks and electrical issues	Yes	No	NA	Comments
• Are electrical cords and plugs free from cracks, fraying, or other damage?				
• Are power strips overloaded?				
• Is electricity being used near a water source?				
• Are flammable chemicals and supplies stored according to manufacturers' guidelines?				
• Are combustibles (e.g., paper, cardboard, cloth, flammable chemicals) away from heat sources?				

Fire containment and evacuation strategies	Yes	No	NA	Comments
• Are building diagrams posted on walls indicating exit routes (two or more), fire alarms, and fire extinguishers?				
• Are exit routes uncluttered?				
• Are exit signs visible and lit?				
• Are fire doors unblocked and able to be closed in an emergency?				
• Are interior rooms available for severe storms?				
• Are smoke detectors located throughout the building?				
• Are fire alarms available?				
• Are fire extinguishers available and checked routinely (per the facility's policy)?				
• Are flammable products (e.g., oxygen tanks, chemicals) stored along the exit routes?				

Based on your observations, summarize your findings.

If risks are present, create a list of issues that need to be addressed. Describe what needs to be done for each risk.

Procedure 13.5   Participate in a Mock Exposure Event

Name _____   **Date** _____   **Score** _____

Tasks: Demonstrate self-awareness in an emergency situation. Participate in a mock exposure event and document specific steps taken. Recognize the physical and emotional effects on individuals involved in an emergency situation.

Scenario: You and Beth are in the autoclave room and two chemicals spill, creating toxic fumes. Beth is having trouble breathing. The staff, patients, and visitors present include:

Rooms	Staff and Reception Areas
1—Teen and his mother	Reception Area A—Four people waiting
2—Older woman in a wheelchair	Reception Area B—Five people waiting
3—Mother with three little children	
4—Adult female	**Staff**
5—Empty	Tim—In MA station 3
6—An older couple	Rose—At the insurance desk
7—Adult male	Dave and Patty—At the reception desk
8—Empty	Julie Walden, MD—In provider office 1
Procedure room—Empty	Angela Perez, MD—In room 3
	Jean Burke, NP—In room 7

Directions: Create a paper and address the points in the checklist. Use reliable internet resources to research the physical and emotional effects of stress on the body. Include your findings in the paper as indicated in the checklist. Use 1-inch margins, double spacing, and 12-point font. Length should be at least two pages.

Equipment and Supplies:
- Paper
- Pen
- Floor map (see Figure 13.11 in the textbook)
- Computer with internet access

Standard: Complete the procedure and all critical steps with a minimum score of 85% within two attempts (*or as indicated by the instructor*).

Scoring: Divide the points earned by the total possible points. Failure to perform a critical step, indicated by an asterisk (*), results in grade no higher than an 84% (*or as indicated by the instructor*).

Steps:	Point Value	Attempt 1	Attempt 2
1. Using the scenario, describe how you would handle the emergency exposure situation with Beth. • Identify four steps a medical assistant could take to demonstrate self-awareness while responding to this emergency situation. • Describe exposure control mechanisms or how you might limit the exposure to other people once you remove Beth from the room.	15*		

Principles of Pharmacology

chapter

14

CAAHEP Competencies	Assessment
I.C.11.a. Identify the classifications of medications including: indications for use	Certification Preparation – 9; Workplace Applications – 1; Internet Activities – 3e
I.C.11.b. Identify the classifications of medications including: desired effects	Certification Preparation – 10; Workplace Applications – 1; Internet Activities – 3f
I.C.11.c. Identify the classifications of medications including: side effects	Workplace Applications – 2; Internet Activities – 3h
I.C.11.d. Identify the classifications of medications including: adverse reactions	Workplace Applications – 2; Internet Activities – 3i
IV.C.2. Define the function of dietary supplements	Skills and Concepts – C. 3
ABHES Competencies	**Assessment**
1. General Orientation d. List the general responsibilities and skills of the medical assistant	Skills and Concepts – A. 1-2
1.f. Comply with federal, state, and local health laws and regulations as they relate to healthcare settings	Skills and Concepts – C. 6-7, 9, 11
6. Pharmacology a. Identify drug classification, usual dose, side effects and contraindications of the top most commonly used medications.	Workplace Applications – 1-2; Internet Activities – 3
6.c. 1) Identify parts of prescriptions	Skills and Concepts – F. 2-3
6.c. 2) Identify appropriate abbreviations that are accepted in prescription writing	Abbreviations – 16, 18-24, 27-48; Procedure 14.1
6.c. 3) Comply with legal aspects of creating prescriptions, including federal and state laws	Skills and Concepts – F. 4-6; Procedure 14.1
6.d. Properly utilize the Physician's Desk Reference (PDR), drug handbooks, and other drug references to identify a drug's classification, usual dosage, usual side effects, and contraindications	Internet Activities – 3

VOCABULARY REVIEW

Using the word pool on the right, find the correct word to match the definition. Write the word on the line after the definition.

Group A

1. The study of drug absorption, distribution, metabolism, and excretion in the body _____

2. The study of the properties, actions, and uses of drugs _____

3. A drug that reduces or eliminates pain _____

4. A drug that destroys or inhibits the growth of bacteria _____

5. Unpleasant effects of a drug in addition to the desired or therapeutic effect _____

6. A drug that prevents or alleviates heart arrhythmias _____

7. Harmful and deadly effects of a medication that can develop due to the buildup of medication or byproducts in the body _____

8. A substance (i.e., medication or chemical) that prevent the clotting of blood _____

9. A substance that inhibits the growth of microorganisms on living tissue _____

10. The means by which a drug enters the body _____

Word Pool
- antiarrhythmic
- anticoagulant
- antiseptic
- antibiotic
- analgesic
- side effects
- pharmacology
- toxicity
- route
- pharmacokinetics

Group B

1. Medications that are administered in an inactive form _____

2. A series of chemical processes whereby enzymes change drugs in the body _____

3. Tissues that slowly release the drug into the bloodstream and keep the blood levels from decreasing too rapidly _____

4. A medication that prevents or reduces inflammation _____

5. The movement of metabolites out of the body _____

6. The movement of absorbed drug from the blood to the body tissues _____

7. Route of administration where the drug is placed under the tongue to dissolve _____

8. Route of administration where the drug is placed between the cheek and the gums to dissolve _____

9. The movement of drug from the site of administration to the bloodstream _____

10. Route of medication where the medication is injected just below the skin _____

Word Pool
- antiinflammatory
- reservoirs
- excretion
- absorption
- distribution
- metabolism
- prodrugs
- buccal
- sublingual
- subcutaneous

Group C

1. A medication that slows down the cell's activity _____
2. Byproducts of drug metabolism _____
3. A medication that increases the cell's activity _____
4. Desired effects _____
5. A higher initial dose of medication _____
6. A medication that kills cells or disrupts parts of cells _____
7. Unexpected or life-threatening reaction _____
8. Medical doctors who have been specially trained to diagnose and treat patients with mental, emotional, and behavioral conditions _____
9. A disease that occurs when a person cannot stop or limit the use of a drug, even after negative consequences have been experienced _____
10. Is reached when the blood concentration of a medication is high enough for the therapeutic effect to occur _____

Word Pool
- psychiatrists
- loading dose
- destroying
- adverse reaction
- metabolites
- addiction
- depressing
- stimulating
- therapeutic range
- therapeutic effects

Group D

1. Information that appears on the drug label and addresses serious or life-threatening risks _____
2. Comparing a document with another document to ensure that they are consistent _____
3. Conditions or diseases for which the drug is used _____
4. A medication order given in person or over the phone _____
5. Directions given by a provider for a specific medication to be administered to a patient _____
6. Reasons or conditions that make administration of the drug improper or undesirable _____
7. A written order by a provider to the pharmacist _____
8. An identifier assigned by the Centers for Medicare and Medicaid Services (CMS) that classifies the healthcare provider by license and medical specialties _____
9. Indicates the greatest amount of medication a person should have within a 24-hour period _____
10. Physical characteristics of a medication (e.g., tablet and suspension) _____

Word Pool
- contraindications
- indication
- form
- verbal order
- medication order
- prescription
- National Provider Identifier
- maximum dosage
- boxed warning
- reconciling

ABBREVIATIONS

Write out what each of the following abbreviations stands for.

1. IV _____

2. ID _____

3. NAS _____

4. subcut _____

5. PO _____

6. ung _____

7. soln, sol. _____

8. cap _____

9. tinct _____

10. IM _____

11. C _____

12. F _____

13. m _____

14. cm _____

15. mm _____

16. tab(s) _____

17. kg _____

18. g _____

19. mg _____

20. mcg _____

21. gr _____

22. gtt(s) _____

23. L _____

24. mL _____

25. lb _____

26. fl oz _____

27. qt _____

28. pt _____

29. Tbs, tbsp _____

30. tsp _____

31. AM, a.m. _____

32. PM, p.m. _____

33. pc _____

34. ac _____

35. ad lib _____

36. d _____

37. noc, noct _____

38. hr, h _____

39. $\bar{p}$ _____

40. min _____

41. qh _____

42. prn _____

43. q4h _____

44. q6h _____

45. qam _____

46. tid _____

47. bid _____

48. qid _____

49. STAT _____

50. ASA _____

51. K _____

52. Fe _____

53. NS _____

54. MOM _____

55. NSAID _____

56. PPD _____

57. OTC _____

58. aq _____

59. med _____

60. NKA _____

61. NKDA _____

62. NPO _____

63. $\overline{aa}$ _____

64. $\overline{c}$ _____

65. $\overline{s}$ _____

66. pt _____

67. qs _____

68. Rx _____

69. Sig _____

70. VO _____

71. x _____

SKILLS AND CONCEPTS

Answer the following questions. Write your answer on the line or in the space provided.

A. Introduction

1. Explain why medical assistants need to know about medications. _____

_____

_____

2. Describe what medical assistants need to know about medications. _____

_____

_____

B. Pharmacology Basics

1. List the natural sources of drugs and give one example for each. _____

_____

_____

2. List two advantages to synthetic medications. _____

_____

_____

3. Describe the eight uses of drugs and list one example for each use. _____

_____

_____

_____

_____

_____

4. Describe the four parts of pharmacokinetics. _____

_____

_____

_____

_____

5. Describe the effect of the blood-brain barrier to the distribution of medication. _____

_____

6. Describe why only limited medications can be given to a woman who is pregnant. _____

_____

_____

7. Explain why different routes affect the dose of medication given. _____

_____

_____

_____

_____

8. _____ are medications that are administrated in an inactive form and change into the active form during the metabolic process.

9. Where does most drug metabolism occur? What populations have issues metabolizing medications and are at risk for toxicity?

_____

_____

_____

10. Most metabolites are excreted through the _____ and _____.

11. Describe why medications are limited when a female is breastfeeding her baby. _____

_____

_____

12. List all ways drugs are excreted by the body. _____

_____

13. What three populations are at risk for the buildup of metabolic drug byproducts in the body?_____

_____

14. Describe the four main drug actions._____

_____

_____

_____

_____

15. _____ is the study of how genetic factors influence a person's metabolic response to
a specific medication.

16. Describe six factors that influence drug action. _____

_____

_____

_____

_____

17. Explain why a provider may prescribe a loading dose. Your answer should also include the advantage
of giving a loading dose of medication.

_____

_____

18. _____ occurs when a person develops antibodies against a specific drug.

19. _____ is extreme hypersensitivity to a specific drug (antigen) and can cause life-
threatening symptoms.

20. List four symptoms of anaphylaxis._____

_____

_____

_____

21. _____ is a peculiar response to a certain drug.

22. When prior doses of medications are not excreted before the next dose is given,
_____can occur.

23. The buildup of medication or byproducts in the body can lead to _____, which is
harmful and possibly fatal.

C. Drug Legislation and the Ambulatory Care Setting

1. Describe the activities *prescribe, administer,* and *dispense.* Include who can perform each of these activities.

    _____

    _____

    _____

    _____

2. Describe the Food, Drug, and Cosmetic Act. Who enforces the act? _____

    _____

    _____

3. Define the function of dietary supplements. _____

    _____

    _____

4. Describe the Controlled Substance Act. Who enforces the act?_____

    _____

    _____

    _____

5. Briefly describe the schedule of controlled substances. _____

    _____

    _____

6. What is the DEA registration number? How long is it good for? _____

    _____

    _____

7. Discuss how controlled substances are to be stored._____

    _____

    _____

    _____

8. Discuss storage of medications (in general)._____

    _____

    _____

    _____

9. Discuss the importance of keeping inventory records of controlled substances. Your answer should also include the importance of reconciling the log and the length of time the logs need to be kept.

   _____

   _____

   _____

   _____

10. What is meant by *diversion* of controlled substances? _____

    _____

    _____

11. If a medical assistant suspects the diversion of controlled substances, discuss what must occur. _____

    _____

    _____

    _____

D. Drug Names

1. The _____ name or _____ name is assigned by the manufacturer and no other company can use that name.

2. The _____ name is assigned by the U.S. Adopted Name Council.

3. The _____ name represents the exact formula of the medication.

4. The _____ name is used to list the medication in the U.S. Pharmacopeia and in the National Formulary (USP-NP).

5. Two companies make the exact same medication. What names would both companies use? What name(s) would be unique for each company?

   _____

   _____

   _____

E. Drug Reference Information

1. Name resources that can be used to learn more about medications. _____

   _____

   _____

   _____

2. Define the following terms.

    a. Dosage _____

    _____

    b. Indication _____

    _____

    c. Contraindications _____

    _____

    d. Precautions _____

    _____

    e. Adverse reactions _____

    _____

    f. Interactions _____

    _____

    g. Action _____

    _____

F. Types of Medication Orders

1. What information must the provider give for a medication order? _____

    _____

    _____

2. Describe the four parts of a prescription. _____

    _____

    _____

3. List the information that must be included for all prescriptions. _____

    _____

    _____

    _____

    _____

4. Describe how prescriptions for schedule II/IIN medications are handled. _____

    _____

    _____

5. Describe how prescriptions for schedule III/III N and IV medications are handled. _____

    _____

    _____

    _____

6. Describe how prescriptions for schedule V medications are handled. _____

    _____

    _____

    _____

CERTIFICATION PREPARATION

Circle the correct answer.

1. The rate of medication absorption is influenced by the
    a. blood flow to the absorption area.
    b. route.
    c. conditions at the site of the absorption.
    d. all of the above.

2. Which statement is true regarding metabolism?
    a. Most drug metabolism occurs in the liver.
    b. Young children, older adults, and those with kidney disease have issues metabolizing medications.
    c. Prodrugs change to inactive forms of drugs during metabolism.
    d. a and c

3. _____ means one drug reduces or blocks the effect of another drug.
    a. Toxicity
    b. Synergism
    c. Antagonism
    d. Potentiation

4. _____ means one drug increases the effect of the second drug.
    a. Toxicity
    b. Synergism
    c. Antagonism
    d. Potentiation

5. _____ means to give a prescribed dose of medication to a patient.
    a. Dispense
    b. Administer
    c. Prescribe
    d. Treatment

6. What is the classification of amoxicillin?
    a. Analgesic
    b. Antianxiety
    c. Antibiotic
    d. Antidepressant

7. What is the classification of atenolol?
    a. Antianxiety
    b. Anticonvulsant
    c. Antidepressant
    d. Antihypertensive

8. What is the classification of albuterol?
    a. Cholesterol-lowering agent
    b. Bronchodilator
    c. Corticosteroid
    d. Antihypertensive

9. Which classification of medication increases urinary output and lowers blood pressure?
    a. Laxative
    b. Corticosteroid
    c. Antihypertensive
    d. Diuretic

10. What is the action of an antiemetic?
    a. Treats depression
    b. Reduces nausea and vomiting
    c. Treats bacterial infections
    d. Reduces blood glucose level

WORKPLACE APPLICATIONS

1. Using Table 14.4, Information on Commonly Prescribed Medications, complete the table. Identify the indications for use and the desired effects for the medication classifications listed.

Medication Classification	Indications for Use	Desired Effects
Analgesics		
Antianxiety		
Antiarrhythmic		
Antibiotics		
Anticoagulants		
Anticonvulsants		
Antidepressants		
Antihistamines		
Antihyperglycemics (noninsulin)		
Antihypertensives		
Antiplatelets		
Bronchodilators		
Cholesterol-lowering agents		
Corticosteroids (oral)		
Diuretics		
Muscle relaxants		
Stimulants		

2. Using Table 14.4, Information on Commonly Prescribed Medications, complete the table. Identify the two side effects and two adverse reactions for the following medication classifications.

Class	Generic Name	Side Effects	Adverse Reaction
Analgesics (narcotic)	hydrocodone/ acetaminophen		
Anti-Alzheimer	memantine		
Antianxiety (benzodiazepines)	alprazolam		
Antiarrhythmics	digoxin		
Antibiotics (penicillin)	amoxicillin		
Anticoagulants	warfarin		
Anticonvulsants	gabapentin		
Antidepressant (SSRIs)	escitalopram		
Antihistamines	promethazine		
Antihyperglycemics	metformin		
Antihypertensive	valsartan		
Bronchodilators	albuterol		
Cholesterol-lowering agents	atorvastatin		
Diuretics	furosemide		
Proton-pump inhibitors	omeprazole		

INTERNET ACTIVITIES

1. Using online resources, identify four reliable websites that can be used for medication information. Cite the websites.

2. Using the internet, research the Prescribers' Digital Reference website (www.pdr.net) or the MedlinePlus website (medlineplus.gov). Summarize the following points in a paper, PowerPoint Presentation, or in a poster.
   a. What types of drug information are available?
   b. How can a medical assistant use this website?
   c. What resources are available on this website?

3. Using appropriate online drug reference resources, research one medication from 12 different classifications listed in Table 14.3. The medications should not be listed on Table 14.4. Cite your references. In a paper, PowerPoint presentation, or poster, address the following points for each of the 12 medications:
   a. Generic name
   b. Trade names (in the U.S. only)
   c. Usual adult dose
   d. Classification
   e. Indication for use
   f. Desired effects
   g. Contraindications (list two or more)
   h. Side effects (list five or more)
   i. Adverse reactions (list three or more)

Procedure 14.1 Prepare a Prescription

Name _____ Date _____ Score _____

Tasks: Prepare prescriptions using a prescription refill protocol. Use approved abbreviations.

Scenario: You received a call from Noemi Rodriguez (DOB 11/04/1971). She is requesting refills on three of her prescriptions from Jean Burke, NP. She saw Jean Burke 10 months ago. Noemi has NKA. She is doing well with the prescriptions and has no concerns. You determine it is time for refills. Her prescriptions include Coumadin 5 mg, 1 tablet orally daily; Tenormin 50 mg, 1 tablet orally daily; and Plendil 5 mg, 1 tablet orally daily.

Prescription Refill Protocol
Walden-Martin Family Medicine Clinic

Description: A Certified Medical Assistant (CMA) can refill current hypertensive medications that fall within the guidelines of this protocol.

Step 1	Step 2	
For medications to be refilled, the following points need to be addressed.	**Qualifying Medications**	**Prescription Refill**
• Has the person seen the provider within the last year? • Is the prescription for a hypertensive, hyperlipidemia, or hyperthyroidism medication, a current prescription? • Is the person free of concerns or complications due to the medication? • Is it time for a refill? (The medical assistant must verify that it is time for a refill.) If the answers to the above questions are all YES, then proceed to Step 2. If any of the answers to the above questions are NO, then schedule the person for an appointment with the provider.	amlodipine amlodipine/benazepril atenolol atenolol/chlorthalidone benazepril captopril diltiazem enalapril felodipine fosinopril irbesartan isradipine lisinopril losartan nifedipine quinapril ramipril	Extend the current prescription for 6 months. Instruct patient that in 6 months: • A visit to the provider will be required • Blood pressure reading will be required • Lab work may be required

Equipment and Supplies:
- SimChart for the Medical Office (SCMO) or paper prescriptions (Work Product 14.1) and pen
- Prescription refill protocol
- Drug reference book or online resource

Standard: Complete the procedure and all critical steps in _____ minutes with a minimum score of 85% within two attempts (*or as indicated by the instructor*).

Scoring: Divide the points earned by the total possible points. Failure to perform a critical step, indicated by an asterisk (*), results in grade no higher than an 84% (*or as indicated by the instructor*).

Time: Began_____ Ended_____ Total minutes: _____

Walden-Martin Family Medical Clinic
1234 AnyStreet, AnyTown, AnyState, 12345
Phone: 123-123-1234 Fax: 123-123-5678

Jean Burke NP, Family Nurse Practitioner

Patient: _____ DOB: _____

Address: _____ Date: _____

R Route:

Sig:

Disp:

Refills:

☐   Generics permitted

_____
Jean Burke, NP
NPI#:1234567891

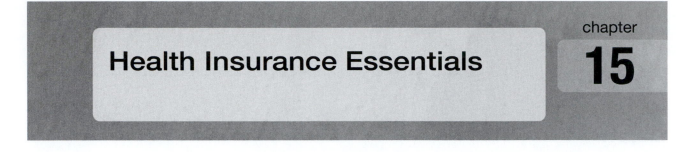

Health Insurance Essentials

chapter

15

CAAHEP Competencies	Assessment
VIII.C.1.a. Identify: types of third party plans	Skills and Concepts – B. 1
VIII.C.2. Outline managed care requirements for patient referral	Skills and Concepts – B. 4
VIII.C.3.a. Describe processes for: verification of eligibility for services	Skills and Concepts – D. 2
VIII.C.3.c. Describe processes for: preauthorization	Skills and Concepts – D. 3, 4
ABHES Competencies	**Assessment**
5. Human Relations c. Assist the patient in navigating issues and concerns that may arise (i.e., insurance policy information, medical bills, and physician/provider orders)	Case Scenario 2

VOCABULARY REVIEW

Using the word pool on the right, find the correct word to match the definition. Write the word on the line after the definition.

Group A

1. A set dollar amount that the policyholder must pay before the insurance company starts to pay for services _____

2. Poor, needy, impoverished _____

3. The amount paid or to be paid by the policyholder for coverage under the contract, usually in periodic installments _____

4. Services provided to help prevent certain illnesses or that lead to an early diagnosis _____

5. When the policyholder pays a certain percentage of the bill and the insurance company pays the rest _____

6. A formal request for payment from an insurance company for services provided _____

7. A written agreement between two parties, in which one party (the insurance company) agrees to pay another party (the patient) if certain specified circumstances occur _____

8. Services that are necessary to improve the patient's current health _____

9. A set dollar amount that the policyholder must pay for each office visit _____

10. The person responsible for the payment of the premium _____

Word Pool
- policy
- premium
- subscriber
- deductible
- coinsurance
- copayment
- claim
- medically necessary
- preventive care
- indigent

Group B

1. Government insurance plan for dependents of military personnel
   _____
2. Those covered by Medicare; a designated person who receives funds from an insurance policy _____
3. Government insurance plan for employees who are injured or become ill due to work-related issues _____
4. Low-income Medicare patients who qualify for Medicaid for their secondary insurance _____
5. Government insurance plan for those age 65 or older
   _____
6. A list of fixed prices for services _____
7. Government insurance plan for surviving spouses and dependent children of veterans who died in the line of duty
   _____
8. A document sent by the insurance company to the provider and the patient explaining the allowed charge amount, the amount reimbursed for services, and the patient's financial responsibilities
   _____
9. Government insurance plan for those with low income
   _____
10. A system used to determine how much providers should be paid for services provided; used by Medicare and many other health insurance companies _____

Word Pool
- Medicare
- Medicaid
- TRICARE
- Civilian Health and Medical Program of the Veterans Administration
- Workers' compensation
- beneficiary
- resource-based relative value scale
- explanation of benefits
- fee schedule
- Qualified Medicare Beneficiaries

Group C

1. In charge of coordinating the patient's care
   _____
2. When the patient has authorized the insurance company to make the payment directly to the provider _____
3. An approved list of physicians, hospitals, and other providers
   _____
4. An organization that processes claims and provides administrative services for another organization
   _____
5. A process required by some insurance carriers in which the provider obtains permission to perform certain procedures or services _____
6. An online marketplace where you can compare and buy individual health insurance plans _____
7. The primary care provider who is in charge of a patient's treatment _____
8. The amount paid for a medical service in a geographic area based on what providers in the area usually charge for the same or similar service _____
9. Insurance plan funded by a large company or organization for their own employees _____
10. An order from a primary care provider for the patient to see a specialist or get certain medical services _____

Word Pool
- self-funded plan
- third-party administrator
- health insurance exchange
- assignment of benefits
- usual, customary, and reasonable
- primary care provider
- referral
- preauthorization
- gatekeeper
- provider network

9. List the services covered by workers' compensation plans._____

_____

_____

_____

_____

10. Private health insurance plans are obtained from two sources. List those sources._____

_____

B. Health Insurance Models

1. Traditional health insurance plans are also referred to as _____ plans.

2. For each of the following managed care plans, describe the deductible, coinsurance, and copayment requirements:

   a. Health maintenance organization (HMO): _____

   _____

   _____

   _____

   _____

   _____

   b. Preferred provider organization (PPO):_____

   _____

   _____

   _____

   _____

   _____

   c. Exclusive provider organization (EPO):_____

   _____

   _____

   _____

   _____

   _____

3. A(n) _____ is a review of individual cases by a committee to make sure services are medically necessary and to study how providers use medical care resources.

4. Describe the managed care requirements for a patient referral. _____

_____

_____

_____

_____

C. Participating Provider Contracts

1. A(n) _____ is a healthcare provider who enters into a contract with a specific insurance company or program and agrees to accept the contracted fee schedule.

2. The _____ is the maximum that third-party payers will pay for a procedure or service.

D. The Medical Assistant's Role

1. One of the medical assistant's responsibilities is verifying eligibility. Describe the processes available for the verification of eligibility for services.

_____

_____

_____

2. Describe how the patient's insurance eligibility is confirmed. _____

_____

_____

_____

3. What items should the medical assistant gather when using the paper method to obtain a precertification for a service or procedure?

_____

_____

_____

4. Describe the processes for precertification using the paper method. What does the medical assistant need to do?

_____

_____

_____

E. Other Types of Insurance

1. Match the types of insurance benefits with their description.

_____ Disability

_____ Liability insurance

_____ Life insurance

_____ Long-term care insurance

a. Provides payment of a specified amount upon the insured's death
b. Covers a continuum of broad-range maintenance and health services to chronically ill, disabled, or mentally disabled individuals
c. A form of insurance that provides income replacement if the patient has a non-work–related injury
d. Often includes benefits for medical expenses related to traumatic injuries and lost wages payable to individuals who are injured in the insured person's home or in an automobile accident

CERTIFICATION PREPARATION

Circle the correct answer.

1. A policy that covers a number of people under a single master contract issued to the employer or to an association with which they are affiliated and that is not self-funded is usually called
   a. a group policy.
   b. an individual policy.
   c. a government plan.
   d. a self-insured plan.

2. The maximum amount of money third-party payers will pay for a specific procedure or service is called the
   a. benefit.
   b. allowed amount.
   c. allowable service.
   d. incurred amount.

3. A provider who enters into a contract with an insurance company and agrees to certain rules and regulations is called a _____ provider.
   a. paying
   b. physician
   c. participating
   d. none of the above

4. A review of individual cases by a committee to make sure that services are medically necessary and to study how providers use medical care resources is called a(n)
   a. credentialing committee review.
   b. peer review committee evaluation.
   c. utilization review.
   d. audit committee review.

5. Which type of HMO model consists of physicians with separately owned practices who formally organize into a group but continue to practice in their own offices?
   a. Staff model
   b. Independent practice association
   c. Group model
   d. None of the above

6. Which individuals would not normally be eligible for Medicare?
   a. A 66-year-old retired woman
   b. A blind teenager
   c. A 23-year-old recipient of Temporary Assistance for Needy Families (TANF)
   d. A person on dialysis

7. Which expenses would be paid by Medicare Part B?
   a. Inpatient hospital charges
   b. Hospice services
   c. Home healthcare charges
   d. Physician's office visits

8. A type of insurance that protects workers from loss of wages after an industrial accident that happened on the job is called
   a. an individual policy.
   b. workers' compensation.
   c. unemployment insurance.
   d. disability insurance.

9. A payment method in which providers are paid for each individual enrolled in a plan, regardless of whether the person sees the provider that month, is called a _____ plan.
   a. capitation
   b. self-insured
   c. managed care
   d. fee-for-service

10. What should the medical assistant always verify prior to the patient's appointment?
    a. Eligibility
    b. Benefits and exclusions
    c. Effective date of insurance
    d. All of the above

WORKPLACE APPLICATIONS

1. After reading the following paragraph, fill the blanks in the statements.

   The medical assistant's tasks related to health insurance processing are initiated when the patient encounters the provider by appointment, as a walk-in, or in the emergency department or hospital. To complete insurance billing and coding properly, the medical assistant must perform the following tasks:

   a. Obtain information from the patient and/or the guarantor, including _____ and _____ data.

   b. Verify the patient's _____ for insurance payment with the insurance carrier or carriers, as well as insurance _____, exclusions, and whether _____ is required to refer patients to specialists or to perform certain services or procedures such as surgery or diagnostic tests.

   c. Obtain _____ for referral of the patient to a specialist or for special services or procedures that require advance permission.

2. Julia Berkley has just gotten a new insurance policy and is struggling with all of the terminology she is seeing in her policy. She would like you to explain just what *premium, deductible, coinsurance,* and *copayment* really mean.

   _____

   _____

   _____

   _____

INTERNET ACTIVITIES

1. Using online resources, research TRICARE and CHAMPVA. Create a poster presentation, a PowerPoint presentation, or write a paper summarizing your research. Include the following points in your project:
   a. Describe both TRICARE and CHAMPVA
   b. List who is eligible for TRICARE and who is eligible for CHAMPVA
   c. Explain what is involved when a provider participates in TRICARE

2. Using online resources, research Preferred Provider Organizations (PPO). Create a poster presentation, a PowerPoint presentation, or write a paper summarizing your research. Include the following points in your project:
   a. Description what a PPO is
   b. List the ranges for deductibles and coinsurance amounts found
   c. Explain how a PPO is different from an HMO
   d. Describe why a patient might want to have a PPO policy instead of traditional insurance

VOCABULARY REVIEW

Using the word pool on the right, find the correct word to match the definition. Write the word on the line after the definition.

Group A

1. The relative frequency of deaths in a specific population

    _____

2. Information about a patient's diagnosis or diagnoses that has been taken from the medical documentation _____

3. Any meeting between a patient and a healthcare provider

    _____

4. Radiology, pathology, and laboratory reports

    _____

5. The study of the causes or origin of diseases

    _____

6. The branch of medicine dealing with the incidence, distribution, and control of disease in a population _____

7. Determining the cause of a condition, illness, disease, injury, or congenital defect _____

8. Accepted healthcare services that are appropriate for the evaluation and treatment of a disease, condition, illness, or injury and are consistent with the applicable standard of care

    _____

9. Software that will apply diagnostic or procedure codes to medical conditions or procedures _____

10. To make repayment for an expense or a loss incurred

    _____

Word Pool
- diagnosis
- reimbursement
- mortality
- epidemiology
- encounter
- encoder
- diagnostic statement
- ancillary diagnostic services
- medically necessary
- etiology

Group B

1. A mental disorder in which the individual experiences a progressive loss of memory, personality alterations, confusion, loss of touch with reality, and stupor _____

2. Patient's chief complaint or statements about why the patient is seeking medical care _____

3. Developing slowly and lasting for a long time, generally 3 or more months _____

4. Suggest that it should not be used _____

5. An abnormal condition resulting from a previous disease _____

6. A document used to capture the services/procedures and diagnoses for a patient visit _____

7. The quality or state of being specific _____

8. A statement in the patient's own words that describes the reason for the visit _____

9. Abbreviations, punctuation, symbols, instructional notations, and related entities _____

10. Collecting important information from the health record _____

Word Pool
- chronic
- specificity
- conventions
- sequela
- dementia
- abstract
- encounter form
- chief complaint
- contraindicate
- subjective findings

Group C

1. Progressive loss of transparency of the lens of the eye _____

2. The signs and symptoms of a disease _____

3. The period from the last month of pregnancy to 5 months postpartum _____

4. Imminently threatening _____

5. First 6 weeks after delivery _____

6. The study of body tissues _____

7. Any measurable indicators found during the physical examination _____

8. Pregnancy _____

9. Advanced hypothyroidism in adulthood _____

Word Pool
- objective findings
- manifestation
- cataract
- myxedema
- impending
- histologic
- antepartum
- postpartum
- peripartum

ABBREVIATIONS

Write out what each of the following abbreviations stands for.

1. ICD-10-CM _____

2. CMS _____

3. WHO _____

4. EHR _____

5. HPI _____

6. H&P _____

7. CC _____

8. HIV _____

9. AIDS _____

10. DM _____

SKILLS AND CONCEPTS

Answer the following questions. Write your answer on the line or in the space provided.

A. What Is Diagnostic Coding?

1. Define *medically necessary* and explain how it applies to diagnostic coding. Give an example. _____

_____

_____

_____

_____

B. Getting to Know the ICD-10-CM

1. Fill in the blanks in the following statements with terms from the word bank to describe how to use the most current diagnostic coding classification system.

Word Bank:

code	coding guidelines	character
convention	diagnostic	diagnostic statements
essential modifier	exclusion	ICD-10-CM
main term	Tabular List	

a. Abstract the correct diagnosis from the _____ found in the patient health record.

b. Use the _____ to look up the diagnosis in the Alphabetic Index.

c. Review the _____ under the main term.

d. Choose the correct code based on the _____ statement.

e. Look up the code from the Alphabetic Index in the _____.

f. Check for any _____, _____, inclusion notes, _____ notes, or additional _____ symbol.

g. Assign the final _____ diagnosis code.

2. ICD-10-CM codes can have up to _____ characters. A(n) _____ "x" is used to fill in for positions that don't have characters.

3. What are the seventh characters used for encounter types and what do they indicate? _____

    _____

    _____

    _____

4. Four basic forms of punctuation are used in the Tabular Index. List them and what they are used for.

    _____

    _____

    _____

    _____

    _____

    _____

5. Match the following terms.

    _____ Main terms

    _____ Nonessential modifiers

    _____ Subterms

    _____ Essential modifiers

    a. These terms are indented under the main term; they change the description of the diagnosis in bold type
    b. Appear in bold
    c. Are found after the main term and are enclosed in parentheses
    d. Indented under the essential modifier

6. Review the following diagnostic statements and determine the main term and essential modifier in the Alphabetic Index.

    a. Morgan Smith had an acute myocardial infarction, commonly referred to as a *heart attack*.

        Main Term: _____   Essential Modifier: _____

    b. Georgia Summers went into anaphylactic shock after drinking milk.

        Main Term: _____   Essential Modifier: _____

    c. Roger Costen has benign essential hypertension.

        Main Term: _____   Essential Modifier: _____

    d. Raul Castro has been diagnosed with iron-deficiency anemia.

        Main Term: _____   Essential Modifier: _____

    e. Stephanie Thompson has a urinary tract infection.

        Main Term: _____   Essential Modifier: _____

    f. Mabel Johnson has rheumatoid arthritis.

        Main Term: _____   Essential Modifier: _____

g. Amanda Smith was diagnosed with multiple sclerosis.

Main Term: _____ Essential Modifier: _____

h. Hudson Madison suffered a ruptured abdominal aneurysm.

Main Term: _____ Essential Modifier: _____

i. Don Julius died last week from congestive heart failure.

Main Term: _____ Essential Modifier: _____

j. Betty White has allergic gastroenteritis.

Main Term: _____ Essential Modifier: _____

C. Preparing for Diagnostic Coding

1. The SOAP notes system of documentation divides the information into what four areas?

a. _____

b. _____

c. _____

d. _____

2. To prepare for medical coding, the coder must analyze the patient's health record and _____ the diagnostic statement.

3. Information pertinent to code selection can be abstracted from a variety of medical documents. List the documents where the diagnostic statement may be found.

_____

_____

_____

_____

_____

4. The _____ is the provider's health history evaluation and physical assessment of the patient.

5. The _____ is a statement in the patient's own words that describes why the person is seeking medical attention.

6. The _____ is used for extracting procedure and diagnostic information for patients who underwent surgery.

D. Steps in ICD-10-CM Coding

1. Code the following diagnoses to the highest level of specificity using either the ICD-10-CM coding manual or the TruCode encoder.

   a. Kayla Swift was diagnosed with infectious mononucleosis. _____

   b. Gerald Weaver has osteoarthritis in his right shoulder region. _____

   c. Jeffrey Rush has a personal history of alcoholism. _____

   d. Barry White's alcoholism has caused cirrhosis of the liver without ascites. _____

   e. Frank Emmett had atherosclerosis of the extremities with gangrene. _____

   f. Ginger Chan experienced dermatitis from using facial cosmetics. _____

   g. The Lewises' first child was born with Down syndrome. _____

   h. Lee Anna has experienced painful menstruation during her last three cycles. _____

   i. Gary Stevens was diagnosed with cardiomegaly. _____

   j. Jerry Stein developed Kaposi's sarcoma in his lymph nodes during the final stages of AIDS. _____

   k. Terri Holden attempted suicide for the second time using a handful of lithium. _____

   l. Susan French was stung by a jellyfish while swimming off the coast of Mexico. _____

   m. Riley Brown has acute myocarditis. _____

   n. Ordell Thompson has acute esophagitis. _____

   o. Korney Ralphy was diagnosed with systemic lupus erythematosus. _____

   p. Marcia Radson had a skin condition known as *bullous pemphigoid*, in which blisters form in patches all over her skin. _____

   q. Osteomalacia caused by malnutrition made it impossible for Robbie Hernandez to walk. _____

   r. Henry Casper has oral leukoplakia, which may have been caused by smoking a pipe. _____

   s. Patricia Kielty has had uterine endometriosis for several years and may require a hysterectomy in the future. _____

   t. Robert Bauer dislocated his right shoulder while playing baseball; it was a closed anterior dislocation. _____

CERTIFICATION PREPARATION

Circle the correct answer.

1. Which term defines a malignant neoplasm as the absence of invasion of surrounding tissues?
   a. Primary
   b. Secondary
   c. In situ
   d. Benign

2. Which code will be used for a patient with a history of myocardial infarction with no symptoms but diagnosed by means of an electrocardiogram?
   a. I21
   b. I25.2
   c. I21.3
   d. None of the above

3. Which term applies to the period from the last month of pregnancy to 5 months after giving birth?
   a. Antepartum
   b. Childbirth
   c. Postpartum
   d. Peripartum

4. The abbreviation that is the equivalent of "unspecified" is _____.
   a. NEC
   b. NOS
   c. NOW
   d. NCL

5. If the provider has documented "rule out" in the diagnostic statement, the medical assistant must code what?
   a. Whatever phrase follows "rule out"
   b. Lab results
   c. Signs/symptoms
   d. None of the above

6. A diagnosis is
   a. a third party's opinion of a patient's illness.
   b. determining the cause of a patient's illness.
   c. the process of finding a patient's past medical history.
   d. both b and c.

7. Currently in the United States, the book used for coding diagnoses in physicians' offices is the
   a. Diagnostic Guide for Medicare and Medicaid Services.
   b. Diagnostic Codes for Third-Party Payers.
   c. International Classification of Disease, 10th Edition, Clinical Modifications.
   d. AMA Manual of Essential Diagnostic Codes, Volume 1.

8. Morbidity is the presence of illness or disease, whereas mortality is
   a. the determination of the nature of a disease.
   b. the deaths that occur from a disease.
   c. classification of a disease.
   d. All of the above.

9. In ICD-10, codes longer than three characters always have a decimal point between the
   a. fourth and fifth characters.
   b. fifth and sixth characters.
   c. third and fourth characters.
   d. sixth and seventh characters.

10. In the ICD-10-CM coding system, a lowercase "x" is used
    a. as a placeholder character within a code.
    b. to denote an obsolete code.
    c. as a cross-reference guide.
    d. to indicate the external causes of morbidity.

WORKPLACE APPLICATIONS

1. Dr. Martin has diagnosed Maude Crawford in the past with congestive heart failure and diabetes mellitus type 2 (insulin-dependent, long-term). She comes to the clinic today complaining of chest pain and has a fever of 101.8° F. Code all of these conditions. In which order should these codes be sequenced?

    a. _____
    b. _____
    c. _____
    d. _____
    e. _____

2. Dr. Perez has documented the following for Reuven Ahmad:

    CC: Shortness of breath, chest pain, nausea, and excessive sweating
    DX: 1. probable myocardial infarction, 2. rule out gastroesophageal reflux disease

    What are the correct diagnosis codes for this patient?

    Note to instructors: Remind students that codes may change with updated versions of ICD.

INTERNET ACTIVITIES

1. Using online resources, research diagnostic code encoders. Create a poster presentation, a PowerPoint presentation, or write a paper summarizing your research. Include the following points in your project:
    a. Describe the purpose of an encoder.
    b. List three reasons why a healthcare organization would want to use an encoder for diagnostic coding.
    c. Explain how using an encoder is different than using the ICD-10-CM coding manuals.

2. Using online resources, research the history and development of ICD. Create a poster presentation, a PowerPoint presentation, or write a paper summarizing your research. Include the following points in your project:
    a. Describe the ICD system.
    b. Explain how and why it was originally developed.
    c. List five reasons why ICD-10-CM was developed.

Procedure 16.1   Perform Coding Using the Current ICD-10-CM Manual or Encoder

Name _____   Date _____   Score _____

Task: To perform accurate diagnosis coding using the ICD-10-CM manual or encoder.

Scenario: The encounter form and progress notes both show that the diagnosis for this patient encounter is acute colitis. Locate the most accurate ICD-10-CM code for this diagnostic statement.

Equipment and Supplies:
- ICD-10-CM manual (current year) *or*
- Encoder software such as TruCode

Standard: Complete the procedure and all critical steps in _____ minutes with a minimum score of 85% within two attempts (*or as indicated by the instructor*).

Scoring: Divide the points earned by the total possible points. Failure to perform a critical step, indicated by an asterisk (*), results in grade no higher than an 84% (*or as indicated by the instructor*).

Time: Began_____ Ended_____ Total minutes: _____

Steps:	Point Value	Attempt 1	Attempt 2
Alphabetic Index			
1. Determine and locate the main terms from the diagnostic statement in the Alphabetic Index.	10		
2. Locate the essential modifiers listed under the main term in the Alphabetic Index.	10		
3. Review the conventions, punctuation, and notes in the Alphabetic Index.	10		
4. Choose a tentative code, codes, or code range from the Alphabetic Index that matches the diagnostic statement as closely as possible.	15*		
Tabular List			
5. Look up the codes chosen from the Alphabetic Index in the Tabular List.	10		
6. Review notes, conventions, and the Official Coding Guidelines associated with the code and code description in the Tabular List. a. Review conventions and punctuation. b. Review instructional notations: • *Includes* and *excludes* notes • *Code first, code also,* and *code additional* notes • *and, or,* and *with* statements	10		
7. Verify the accuracy of the tentative code in the Tabular List. a. Make sure all elements of the diagnostic statement are included in the codes selected. b. Make sure the code description does not include anything not documented in the diagnostic statement.	10		
8. Extend the codes to their highest level of specificity (up to the 7th character, if required). If a 7th character is required, and no codes are present for the 4th, 5th, or 6th characters, it is appropriate to use the dummy placeholder X for these positions.	10		

VOCABULARY REVIEW

Using the word pool on the right, find the correct word to match the definition. Write the word on the line after the definition.

Group A

1. An online journal, supported by the AMA, that addresses subjects such as appealing insurance denials, validating coding to auditors, training staff members, and answering day-to-day coding questions _____

2. The use of a lower-level procedure code than is justified _____

3. Pertaining to, involving, or affecting two or both sides _____

4. The regular collection of data to assess whether the correct processes are being performed and desired results are being achieved _____

5. Additional medical documentation required to confirm the need for the use of unlisted, unusual, or newly adopted medical procedures code _____

6. Two-digit numeric codes that report or indicate specific criteria, specific condition, or special circumstance _____

7. The quality or state of being specific _____

8. The use of a higher-level procedure code than is supported in the documentation or medical necessity _____

9. In medical terms, a medical diagnosis or procedure named for the person who discovered it _____

10. The surgical removal of dead, damaged, or infected tissue to improve the function of healthy tissue _____

Word Pool
- performance measurement
- eponym
- specificity
- CPT Assistant
- débridement
- special report
- upcoding
- downcoding
- modifiers
- bilaterally

Group B

1. Concentrates on the chief complaint; it looks at the symptoms, severity, and duration of the problem _____

2. A list of questions related to each organ system designed to uncover potential disease processes _____

3. Includes chief complaint, extended history of present illness, problem-pertinent system review including a review of a limited number of additional systems and pertinent past, family, and/or social histories directly related to the patient's problems

   _____

4. The process of collecting pertinent medical information needed to assign the correct code _____

5. A statement in the patient's own words that describes the reason for the visit _____

6. The relative incidence of disease _____

7. Includes chief complaint, extended history of present illness, ROS that is directly related to the problem or problems identified in the history of the present illness, review of all additional body systems, in addition to complete past, family, and social histories

   _____

8. Special symbols used to provide additional information about specific codes _____

9. Includes symptoms, severity, and duration of the chief complaint, and a review of systems that relate to the chief complaint

   _____

10. Relates to the number of deaths from a given disease

    _____

Word Pool

- conventions
- abstract
- chief complaint
- review of systems
- problem-focused history
- expanded problem-focused history
- detailed history
- comprehensive history
- morbidity
- mortality

Group C

1. An extended examination is performed on the affected body area and related body areas or organ systems

   _____

2. Determine the amount of drug present _____

3. Limited to the affected body area or single system mentioned in the chief complaint _____

4. Each step of the procedure is listed separately

   _____

5. Medical services and procedures performed for the patient before, during, and after a surgical procedure _____

6. A complete multisystem examination is performed or a complete examination of a single organ system _____

7. Based on the type of drug found _____

8. In addition to the limited body area or system, related body areas or organ systems are examined _____

9. Includes services related to prepping the patient for the procedure, performing the procedure, and suturing to complete the procedure _____

10. A nursing healthcare professional who is certified to administer anesthesia _____

Word Pool

- problem-focused examination
- expanded problem-focused examination
- detailed examination
- comprehensive examination
- Certified Registered Nurse Anesthetist
- global services
- bundled code
- unbundled code
- qualitative
- quantitative

ABBREVIATIONS

Write out what each of the following abbreviations stands for.

1. CPT _____

2. HCPCS _____

3. AMA _____

4. EHR _____

5. H&P _____

6. E/M _____

7. POS _____

8. NP _____

9. EP _____

10. ROS _____

11. CRNA _____

12. NCCI _____

13. MRI _____

14. TURP _____

15. ASA _____

16. RVG _____

SKILLS AND CONCEPTS

Answer the following questions. Write your answer on the line or in the space provided.

A. Introduction to the CPT Manual

1. The CPT was developed and is maintained by the _____.

2. The CPT manual is updated every year on _____.

B. Code Categories in the CPT Manual

1. The CPT code is a five-digit code also known as a(n) _____ code.

2. Category II codes are primarily used for _____ and are optional.

3. Category _____ codes are for new experimental procedures or emerging technology.

C. Organization of the CPT Manual

1. The CPT coding manual organizes codes into the Alphabetic Index and the _____.

2. The six sections of the CPT manual include:

   a. _____

   b. _____

   c. _____

   d. _____

   e. _____

   f. _____

D. Unlisted Procedure or Service Code

1. When using an unlisted procedure code, a(n) _____ must be sent with the insurance claim.

E. General CPT Coding Guidelines

1. _____ are found at the beginning of each of the six sections of the CPT coding manual, and the medical assistant refers to them often when coding procedures.

2. Code additions that explain circumstances that alter a provided service or provide additional clarification or detail are called _____.

32. Urine pregnancy test

_____

33. Polio vaccine, intramuscular route

_____

34. Human papillomavirus (HPV) vaccine, nine types, three-dose schedule, intramuscular route

_____

35. Psychotherapy for crisis; first 60 minutes

_____

HCPCS Coding

1. Standard wheelchair

_____

2. Gradient compression stocking below-knee, 40-50 mm Hg each

_____

3. Above-knee, short prosthesis, no knee joint (stubbies), with articulated ankle/foot, dynamically aligned, right leg

_____

4. Disposable contact lens, per lens, one set

_____

5. Ambulance waiting time, 1 hour

_____

CERTIFICATION PREPARATION

Circle the correct answer.

1. The CPT coding manual is updated annually on
   a. January 1.
   b. December 1.
   c. October 1.
   d. June 1.

2. To find the most accurate code, coders use which progression?
   a. Categories, subcategories, sections, subsections
   b. Sections, subsections, categories, subcategories
   c. Sections, categories, subsections, subcategories
   d. Subsections, subcategories, sections, categories

3. The evaluation and management CPT codes are used for insurance reimbursement in the following healthcare settings *except*
   a. medical office.
   b. weight loss clinic.
   c. nursing home.
   d. hospital.

4. Which codes can be used to help measure performance and outcomes?
   a. Category I codes
   b. Category II codes
   c. Category III codes
   d. Both a and b

5. Which section uses the code range between 70000 and 79999?
   a. Anesthesia section
   b. Surgery section
   c. Radiology section
   d. Medicine section

6. When searching the alphabetic index, "humerus" is an example of a(n)
   a. procedure or service.
   b. organ or anatomic site.
   c. condition, illness, or injury.
   d. eponym, synonym, abbreviation, or acronym.

7. Which level of history includes a review of the systems that relate to the chief complaint?
   a. Problem-focused history
   b. Expanded problem-focused history
   c. Detailed history
   d. Comprehensive history

8. Which HCPCS codes range from A4000 to A8999?
   a. Ambulance transport
   b. Medical supplies
   c. Surgical supplies
   d. Both b and c

9. Which modifier indicates a professional component and is used when a separate technician performs the service but the provider reviews the report and makes a diagnosis?
   a. -50
   b. -62
   c. -26
   d. -RT, -LT

10. Which code is assigned to an urgent care facility as the place of service?
    a. 01
    b. 13
    c. 20
    d. 23

WORKPLACE APPLICATIONS

Identify all procedures that need to be coded for billing purposes in the following situations. Using the most current CPT manual or an encoder such as TruCode, determine the correct CPT codes.

1. Monique Jones is a new patient who saw Dr. Walden to report feeling tired all the time. She stated that she was exhausted even after a full 8 hours of sleep at night. Monique said that she did not have much of an appetite and that she had been eating mostly salads and chicken with a bowl of fruit as snacks. She is not overweight, and her blood pressure and other vital signs were normal. Dr. Walden decided to perform a complete blood count, an electrolyte panel, and a lipid panel. She also ordered a urinalysis, an iron-binding capacity, and a vitamin B12 test. The provider asked the patient if she had noticed any blood in her urine or stool, and she denied blood in the urine but did mention she had several episodes of diarrhea. Dr. Walden added an occult blood test and a stool culture to check for pathogens. The physician placed Monique on multivitamin therapy and told her to return in 1 week to discuss her laboratory test results. She spent approximately 30 minutes with Monique, taking a detailed history and performing a detailed examination, making low-complexity medical decisions. Monique scheduled her appointment for the following week and left the clinic.

2. **Diagnosis:** Left cheek laceration
   Procedure: Repair left cheek laceration

   After the patient was prepped with local anesthetic to the left cheek area, the cheek was dressed and draped with Betadine. The 1.7 cm chin laceration of the skin was closed with three interrupted 6-0 silk sutures. Gentamicin ointment was applied to the lacerations and a dressing was placed on the left cheek. The patient tolerated the procedure well.

Comments

CAAHEP Competencies	Step(s)
IX.P.1. Perform procedural coding	Entire procedure

Procedure 17.3 Working with Providers to Ensure Accurate Code Selection

Name _____ Date _____ Score _____

Task: Communicate respectfully and tactfully with medical providers to ensure accurate code selection.

Background: Using tactful communication skills means using good manners as you provide truthful sensitive information to another person, while considering the person's feelings. Tactful communication skills include verbal and nonverbal communication that shows respect, discretion, compassion, honesty, diplomacy, and courtesy. When you use tactful behaviors, you demonstrate professionalism and you preserve relationships by avoiding conflicts and finding common ground.

Many times, the medical coder is the expert on the accurate CPT and ICD code selections. The highest level of specificity must be used when coding so that appropriate reimbursement can occur. It is not uncommon for the medical coder to interact with providers and assist them in understanding the coding process. During these interactions, it is crucial that the medical coder provides the information in a professional, organized, and logical manner. Using tactful communication skills is critical to maintaining a healthy working relationship with the providers.

Scenario: You are a new medical coder for the medical practice. You have been on the job for 6 weeks and have been seeing a trend that charges are being downcoded. The required documentation is present in the health records, but the providers have been selecting less specific codes for the appointment types. Your goal today is to explain to the providers accurate code selection for the appointment types.

Directions: Using the scenario, role-play with two peers, who will play the providers. You need to discuss the importance of selecting the correct code for reimbursement. You need to demonstrate respect during the conversation and utilize tactful communication skills.

Standard: Complete the role-play in _____ minutes with a minimum score of 100% within two attempts (*or as indicated by the instructor*).

Scoring: Divide the points earned by the total possible points. Met competency: 100% (10 points). Not met competency: 0% (0 points).

Time: Began_____ Ended_____ Total minutes: _____

Affective Behavior	*Directions:* Check behaviors observed during the role-play.					
Respect	**Negative, Unprofessional Behaviors**	**Attempt**		**Positive, Professional Behaviors**	**Attempt**	
		1	**2**		**1**	**2**
	Rude, unkind, disrespectful, and/or impolite			Courteous and polite		
	Brief, abrupt; appeared rushed with the conversation			Took time with providers		
	Unconcerned with person's dignity			Maintained person's dignity		
	Poor eye contact			Proper eye contact		
	Negative nonverbal behaviors			Positive nonverbal behaviors		
	Other:			Other:		

13. NUCC _____

14. PAR _____

15. PCMH _____

16. PCP _____

17. POS _____

18. RA _____

19. SSN _____

SKILLS AND CONCEPTS

Answer the following questions. Write your answer on the line or in the space provided.

A. Medical Billing Process

1. List four types of information collected when a patient calls to schedule an appointment.

   a. _____

   b. _____

   c. _____

   d. _____

2. At the time of the appointment, what two things are copied or scanned into the computer? _____

   _____

3. Describe how the patient's insurance eligibility is confirmed. _____

   _____

   _____

   _____

   _____

4. Referring to the information on the ID card, answer the following questions.

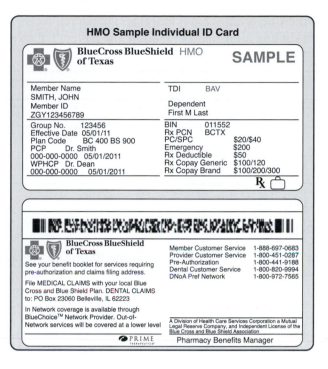

a. What is the member's name? _____

b. What is the member's ID number? _____

c. What is the group number? _____

d. Who is the member's primary care provider (PCP)? _____

e. What is the effective date of the plan? _____

f. What is the deductible for prescriptions (Rx)? _____

g. What is the copay for primary care (PC)? _____

h. What number should the patient call if he has a concern? _____

i. What number should you call if you need to get a preauthorization? _____

j. What number should a healthcare professional working with Dr. Smith call if there is a question about the coverage?

_____

B. Types of Information Found in the Patient's Billing Record

1. The patient's billing record information is often found on the patient registration form. Using Figure 18.1 in the textbook, list the billing information found on the patient registration form.

_____

_____

_____

_____

_____

C. Managed Care Policies and Procedures

1. What items should the medical assistant gather when using the paper method to obtain a precertification for a service or procedure?

_____

_____

_____

_____

_____

2. Describe the processes for precertification using the paper method. What does the medical assistant need to do?

_____

_____

_____

_____

_____

3. Describe the managed care requirements for a patient referral. _____

_____

_____

_____

_____

_____

D. Submitting Claims to Third-Party Payers

1. In your own words, identify the steps for filing a third-party claim. _____

   _____

   _____

   _____

   _____

   _____

   _____

   _____

   _____

E. Generating Electronic Claims

1. Describe the electronic claim form. _____

   _____

   _____

   _____

2. Describe two ways electronic claims can be submitted. _____

   _____

   _____

   _____

3. Describe direct billing. _____

   _____

   _____

   _____

   _____

   _____

   _____

   _____

4. Explain the role of a claims clearinghouse. _____

_____

_____

_____

_____

F. Completing the CMS-1500 Health Insurance Claim Form

1. The medical assistant obtained precertification for a procedure. After the procedure was completed, what are six items needed to complete the CMS-1500 Health Insurance Claim Form?

   a. _____

   b. _____

   c. _____

   d. _____

   e. _____

   f. _____

2. Name the three sections of the claim form.

   a. _____

   b. _____

   c. _____

3. Identify information required to file a third-party claim.

   a. What information must be included in Section 1 of the claim form? _____

   _____

   b. Name 13 pieces of information required in Section 2.

      1. _____

      2. _____

      3. _____

      4. _____

      5. _____

      6. _____

      7. _____

      8. _____

9. _____

10. _____

11. _____

12. _____

13. _____

c. Name 19 pieces of information required in Section 3.

1. _____

2. _____

3. _____

4. _____

5. _____

6. _____

7. _____

8. _____

9. _____

10. _____

11. _____

12. _____

13. _____

14. _____

15. _____

16. _____

17. _____

18. _____

19. _____

G. Accurate Coding to Prevent Fraud and Abuse

1. Differentiate between fraud and abuse. _____

_____

_____

_____

_____

_____

_____

_____

2. What are the possible consequences of coding fraud and abuse?_____

_____

_____

_____

3. In your own words, define *patient-centered medical home* (PCMH). _____

_____

_____

_____

_____

_____

_____

_____

H. Preventing Rejection of a Claim

1. What is the purpose of "claim scrubbers"?_____

_____

_____

_____

_____

I. Checking the Status of a Claim

1. Insurance companies will typically take _____ days to process insurance claims electronically.

2. What information is needed to verify the claim status with insurance company?_____

_____

_____

_____

_____

J. Explanation of Benefits

01/20/20XX

XYZ Insurance Company Explanation of Benefits

Walden-Martin Family Medical Clinic
1234 Anystreet
Anytown, AK 12345-1234

Patient Name	Treatment Dates	CPT Code	Charge Amount	Reason Code	Covered Amount	Deductible Amount	Co-Pay Amount	Paid At	Payment Amount
Yan, Tai	01/06/20XX	99205	132.28	03	125.00	0.00	0.00	80%	100.00
	01/06/20XX	82947	15.00		15.00	0.00	0.00	80%	12.00
	01/06/20XX	86580	11.34		11.34	0.00	0.00	80%	9.07
	Totals		158.62		151.34				121.07
Gomez, Pedro	01/07/20XX	99212	28.55		28.55	0.00	0.00	80%	22.84
	Totals		28.55		28.55				22.84
Green, Jana	01/04/20XX	99203	70.92	03	69.23	0.00	0.00	80%	55.38
	01/04/20XX	71020	40.97	03	34.95	0.00	0.00	80%	27.96
	Totals		111.89		104.18				83.34

Reason Code: 03 Allowed amount per insurance contract

Check No: 56390 $227.25

Using the explanation above answer the following questions:

1. For Tai Yan's office visit, 99205, there is a difference between the Charge Amount and Covered Amount. Based on the reason code supplied what will be done with the difference?

_____

_____

_____

_____

2. How much is Tai Yan responsible for? _____

_____

3. How much will be written off for Jana Green? _____

_____

4. How much is Jana Green responsible for? _____

_____

5. What is the covered amount services provided to Pedro Gomez? _____

_____

K. The Patient's Financial Responsibility

Calculating Coinsurance and Deductible
Use the following information as you answer the following questions.

Patient: Zach Green
Deductible: $750
Coinsurance: 80/20
Patient out-of-pocket expense maximum: $2000

1. During Zach's first visit of the year, he incurred a $500 bill. Who pays this bill?_____

_____

_____

2. During Zach's second visit of the year, he incurred a $450 bill. Describe how much is paid by Zach and the insurance carrier.

_____

_____

3. Zach had surgery, which was his third claim of the year. He had a bill of $5000. Considering the prior visits, what is Zach's portion of this bill and what is the responsibility of the insurance carrier?

_____

_____

_____

_____

4. How much is Zach responsible for so far this year considering his first three visits? _____

_____

_____

_____

CERTIFICATION PREPARATION
Circle the correct answer.

1. To examine claims for accuracy and completeness before they are submitted is to _____ the claims.
   a. correct
   b. audit
   c. revise
   d. reject

2. Block 1 of the CMS-1500 form contains what information?
   a. Patient's name
   b. Insured's name
   c. Type of insurance coverage
   d. Carrier address

3. The patient's name is found in block
   a. 1.
   b. 2.
   c. 3.
   d. 4.

4. CPT codes are found in what block?
   a. 24a
   b. 24b
   c. 24d
   d. 24e

5. Claims with incorrect, missing, or insufficient data are called
   a. clean.
   b. dingy.
   c. incomplete.
   d. dirty.

6. Which is a common reason why insurance claims are rejected?
   a. When a procedure listed is not an insurance benefit
   b. Medical necessity
   c. Preauthorization not obtained
   d. All of the above

7. Which is a fixed amount per visit that is typically paid at the time of medical services?
   a. Copayment
   b. Deductible
   c. Coinsurance
   d. Both a and b

8. Patients sign a(n) _____ of benefits form so that the physician will receive payment for services directly.
   a. release
   b. assignment
   c. turning
   d. sending

9. Claims submitted to a _____ are forwarded to individual insurance carriers.
   a. direct biller
   b. third-party administrator
   c. clearinghouse
   d. post office

10. Electronic data interchange is
    a. transferring data back and forth between two or more entities.
    b. sending information to one insurance carrier.
    c. sending information to one clearinghouse for processing.
    d. None of the above

WORKPLACE APPLICATIONS

1. Sally is the only medical biller in her healthcare agency. One of the two providers orders and performs tests and procedures before getting the needed preauthorizations from the patients' insurance carriers. As a result, the insurance carriers are not covering the claims and the clinic has had to write off thousands of dollars. Discuss how Sally should deal with the situation.

   a. How might she display tactful behavior when communicating with the provider about the third-party requirements?

   _____

   _____

   _____

b. How would you deal with this situation if you were Sally?

_____

_____

_____

2. Christi Brown is meeting with you regarding the bill she received in the mail. When she called to make the appointment, she voiced her confusion about the bill, stating she thought her insurance covered everything. You check her record and see that she met her deductible and now needs to pay 20% of the billed amount. She owes $170. Explain what a deductible and coinsurance are.

_____

_____

_____

INTERNET ACTIVITIES

1. Using online resources, research your insurance carrier or an insurance carrier popular in your area. Research the appeal process for denied claims. Create a poster presentation, a PowerPoint presentation, or write a paper summarizing your research. Include the following points in your project:
   a. Who can start the appeal process?
   b. What steps are involved in the appeal process?
   c. What is the time frame for getting a response to the appeal?

2. Visit http://www.nucc.org and research the resources available on this website. Create a poster presentation, a PowerPoint presentation, or write a paper summarizing your research. Include the following points in your project:
   a. What resources are available for a medical biller on this website?
   b. List three that you think would be most helpful to a medical assistant who does medical billing.
   c. What information is available about the CMS-1500 claim form?
   d. Describe two things you learned from this website.

3. Using online resources, research the most common errors that occur when submitting claims. Create a poster presentation, a PowerPoint presentation, or write a paper summarizing your research. Include the following points in your project:
   a. What are the most common errors?
   b. How can these errors be prevented?
   c. What can a medical assistant do to prevent those errors?

Procedure 18.1   Interpret Information on an Insurance Card

Name _____   Date _____   Score _____

Task: To identify essential information on the health insurance identification (ID) card to confirm copayment obligations and obtain accurate health insurance information for claims submission.

Equipment and Supplies:
- Patient's health insurance ID, both sides (Figure 18.1)

Standard: Complete the procedure and all critical steps in _____ minutes with a minimum score of 85% within two attempts (*or as indicated by the instructor*).

Scoring: Divide the points earned by the total possible points. Failure to perform a critical step, indicated by an asterisk (*), results in grade no higher than an 84% (*or as indicated by the instructor*).

Time: Began_____ Ended_____ Total minutes: _____

Steps:	Point Value	Attempt 1	Attempt 2
1. Review the patient's health insurance ID card and identify the insured on the health insurance ID card. If the patient is different than the insured, then obtain the relationship with the insured and the insured's date of birth and gender.	20*		
2. Identify the insurance plan.	20		
3. Identify the insured's identification number and group number.	20		
4. Identify the patient's copayment, which is due before the appointment. Collect the correct amount.	20		
5. On the back of the health insurance ID card, ensure that a customer service phone number and medical claims address is present.	20		
Total Points	100		

Comments

CAAHEP Competencies	Step(s)
VIII.P.1. Interpret information on an insurance card	Entire procedure
ABHES Competencies	**Step(s)**
7. Administrative Procedures c. Perform billing and collection procedures	Entire procedure

Figure 18.1 Patient's Health Insurance ID Card

HMO Sample Individual ID Card

BlueCross BlueShield HMO
of Texas

SAMPLE

Member Name
SMITH, JOHN
Member ID
ZGY123456789

TDI   BAV

Dependent
First M Last

Group No. 123456	BIN 011552
Effective Date 05/01/11	Rx PCN BCTX
Plan Code BC 400 BS 900	PC/SPC $20/$40
PCP Dr. Smith	Emergency $200
000-000-0000 05/01/2011	Rx Deductible $50
WPHCP Dr. Dean	Rx Copay Generic $100/120
000-000-0000 05/01/2011	Rx Copay Brand $100/200/300

Rx

BlueCross BlueShield
of Texas

See your benefit booklet for services requiring
pre-authorization and claims filing address.

File MEDICAL CLAIMS with your local Blue
Cross and Blue Shield Plan. DENTAL CLAIMS
to: PO Box 23060 Belleville, IL 62223

In Network coverage is available through
BlueChoice™ Network Provider. Out-of-
Network services will be covered at a lower level

Member Customer Service	1-888-697-0683
Provider Customer Service	1-800-451-0287
Pre-Authorization	1-800-441-9188
Dental Customer Service	1-800-820-9994
DNoA Pref Network	1-800-972-7565

A Division of Health Care Services Corporation a Mutual
Legal Reserve Company, and Independent License of the
Blue Cross and Blue Shield Association

PRIME
THERAPEUTICS®

Pharmacy Benefits Manager

Procedure 18.2 Show Sensitivity when Communicating with Patients Regarding Third-Party Requirements

Name _____ Date _____ Score _____

Tasks: Communicate in an assertive, professional manner with a third-party representative. Demonstrate sensitivity through verbal and nonverbal communication when discussing third-party requirements with a patient. Display tactful behavior when communicating with a provider regarding third-party requirements.

Equipment and Supplies:
- Copy of patient's health insurance ID card
- Prescription for new medication

Scenario: Ken Thomas saw Jean Burke N.P. for his asthma today. He was prescribed a fluticasone inhaler 220 mcg and a refill on his albuterol inhaler. When Ken stops at the checkout desk to make a follow-up appointment, he looks concerned. You inquire how you can help him and he states that he is wondering if his new insurance will pick up the fluticasone inhaler. He further explains that he has used it in the past with great results, but he recently switched insurance plans and he is finding it doesn't have the same coverage as his old plan.

- *Role-play #1: You call the insurance company and discuss the coverage with the insurance carrier's representative. The representative tells you that the fluticasone inhaler is not covered for his condition. The representative gave you names of two other inhalers that would be covered.*
    When you ask if the drug would be covered through the exceptions process, the representative indicated that the provider must send a letter indicating the drug is appropriate for the patient's condition because all other drugs covered by the plan have not been effective or those drugs have side effects that may be harmful to the patient or the patient is allergic to the other drugs.
- *Role-play #2: You must explain to Ken, who is upset with his insurance coverage, that he would have to cover the $250 inhaler.*
- *Role-play #3: Ken explains he does not have $250 for the inhaler. He asks what else he should do. You mention the exception process and Ken requests the provider to send a letter. You need to role-play notifying the provider of the third-party requirements.*

Directions: Role-play the scenarios with a peer. The peer will play the part of the insurance representative, the patient, and the provider. You need to be professional and assertive with the insurance representative. When working with the patient, you need to show sensitivity. When communicating with the provider, you need to be professional and tactful.

Standard: Complete the procedure and all critical steps in _____ minutes with a minimum score of 85% within two attempts (*or as indicated by the instructor*).

Scoring: Divide the points earned by the total possible points. Failure to perform a critical step, indicated by an asterisk (*), results in grade no higher than an 84% (*or as indicated by the instructor*).

Time: Began_____ Ended_____ Total minutes: _____

Steps:	Point Value	Attempt 1	Attempt 2
1. Obtain a copy of the patient's health insurance ID card and the prescription for the new medication.	10		
2. Review the insurance card for coverage information and the phone number for providers.	20		

Scenario: Role-play #1 with a peer. The peer will be the insurance representative. 3. Contact the insurance company and clearly state the patient's information, the patient's question, and the new medication. Write down information provided by the representative.	**10***		
4. Demonstrate professionalism through verbal communication skills, by stating a respectful, assertive, clear, organized message while pronouncing medical terminology and medications correctly. *(Refer to the Checklist for Affective Behaviors - Respect)*	**10***		
Scenario: Role-play #2 with a peer. The peer will be the patient. 5. Explain to the patient the message from the insurance representative using language that can be understood by the patient. *(Refer to the Checklist for Affective Behaviors - Respect and Sensitivity)*	**10***		
6. Demonstrate sensitivity to the patient by paying attention to and responding appropriately to the patient's nonverbal body language and verbal message. *(Refer to the Checklist for Affective Behaviors - Respect and Sensitivity)*	**10***		
7. Demonstrate sensitivity to the patient by showing empathy and clarifying that you understand what the patient is stating. Give the patient your full attention during the conversation and reserve judgment. *(Refer to the Checklist for Affective Behaviors - Respect and Sensitivity)*	**10***		
8. Demonstrate sensitivity to the patient by using a pleasant, courteous tone of voice. Use body language to communicate respect (e.g., eye contact if culturally appropriate, keep arms uncrossed and relaxed). *(Refer to the Checklist for Affective Behaviors - Respect and Sensitivity)*	**10***		
Scenario: Role-play #3 with a peer. The peer will be the provider. 9. Demonstrate tactful behavior when explaining the third-party requirements to the provider. *(Refer to the Checklist for Affective Behaviors - Tactful)*	**10***		
Total Points	**100**		

Affective Behavior	**Directions:** Check behaviors observed during the role-play.				
	Negative, Unprofessional Behaviors	**Attempt**		**Positive, Professional Behaviors**	**Attempt**
Respect		**1**	**2**		**1**	**2**
	Rude, unkind			Courteous		
	Disrespectful, impolite			Polite		
	Unwelcoming			Welcoming		
	Brief, abrupt			Took time with patient		
	Unconcerned with person's dignity			Maintained person's dignity		
	Negative nonverbal behaviors			Positive nonverbal behaviors		
	Other:			Other:		

Sensitivity	Distracted; not focused on the other person			Focused full attention on the other person		
	Judgmental attitude; not accepting attitude			Nonjudgmental, accepting attitude		
	Failed to clarify what the person verbally or nonverbally communicated			Used summarizing or paraphrasing to clarify what the person verbally or nonverbally communicated		
	Failed to acknowledge what the person communicated			Acknowledged what the person communicated		
	Rude, discourteous			Pleasant and courteous		
	Disregarded the person's dignity and rights			Maintained the person's dignity and rights		
	Other:			Other:		
Tactful	Improper and/or inappropriate			Proper and appropriate		
	Spoke and/or acted in a manner that was offensive to others; lacked compassion and/or courtesy			Spoke and acted without offending others; showed compassion and courtesy		
	Failed to be sensitive to others when explaining the situation			Explained the situation in a clear and diplomatic way		
	Failed to answer questions; or answers were inappropriate and/or inaccurate			Answered questions appropriately and accurately		
	Other:			Other:		

Grading for Affective Behaviors		Point Value	Attempt 1	Attempt 2
Does not meet Expectation	• Response was insensitive and/or disrespectful. • Student demonstrated more than 2 negative, unprofessional behaviors during the interaction.	0		
Needs Improvement	• Response was insensitive and/or disrespectful. • Student demonstrated 1 or 2 negative, unprofessional behaviors during the interaction.	0		
Meets Expectation	• Response was sensitive and respectful; no negative, unprofessional behaviors observed. • More practice is needed for behavior to appear natural and for student to appear comfortable and at ease.	10		
Occasionally Exceeds Expectation	• Response was sensitive and respectful; no negative, unprofessional behaviors observed. • At times student appeared comfortable and at ease; but more practice is needed for behavior to become natural and consistent with a professional medical assistant.	10		

Always Exceeds Expectation	• Response was sensitive and respectful; no negative, un-professional behaviors observed. • Student's behaviors appeared natural and comfortable. Behaviors are consistent with a professional medical assistant.	10		

Comments

CAAHEP Competencies	Step(s)
VII.P.4 Inform a patient of financial obligations for services rendered	5
VII.A.1. Interact professionally with third party representatives	3-4
VII.A.2 Display sensitivity when requesting payment for services rendered	7
VIII.A.2. Display tactful behavior when communicating with medical providers regarding third party requirements	9
VIII.A.3. Show sensitivity when communicating with patients regarding third party requirements	5-8
ABHES Competencies	**Step(s)**
7. Administrative Procedures c. Perform billing and collection procedures	Entire procedure

Procedure 18.3   Perform Precertification with Documentation

Name _____ Date _____ Score _____

Task: To obtain precertification from a patient's insurance carrier for requested services or procedures.

Equipment and Supplies:
- Paper method: Patient's health record, Prior Authorization (Precertification) Request form, copy of patient's health insurance ID card, a pen
- Electronic method: Electronic health record system such as SimChart for the Medical Office (SCMO)

Scenario: You are working with Dr. Julie Walden at Walden-Martin Family Medical Clinic. Erma Willis (DOB 12/09/19XX) was seen for excessive snoring and Dr. Walden ordered a sleep study. You need to complete a prior authorization/certification form for the sleep study, which will be conducted by Dr. Jim Sandman. You checked and there is a signed release of information form.

Insurance Information	Clinic and Provider Information
Aetna 1234 Insurance Way Anytown, AL 112345-1234 Member ID Number: EW8884910 Group Number: 66574W	Walden-Martin Family Medical Clinic 1234 Anystreet Anytown, AL 12345 Provider: Julie Walden, MD Fax: 123-123-5678 Phone: 123-123-1234 Provider Contact Name: (your name)
Service Information Place: Walden-Martin Family Medicine Clinic Service Requested: Sleep study Starting Service Date: 1 week from today Ending Service Date: 1 week from today Service Frequency: once ICD-10-CM code: R06.83 CPT code: 95807 Not related to an injury or workers' compensation	

Standard: Complete the procedure and all critical steps in _____ minutes with a minimum score of 85% within two attempts (*or as indicated by the instructor*).

Scoring: Divide the points earned by the total possible points. Failure to perform a critical step, indicated by an asterisk (*), results in grade no higher than an 84% (*or as indicated by the instructor*).

Time: Began_____ Ended_____ Total minutes: _____

Steps:	Point Value	Attempt 1	Attempt 2
1. For the paper method, gather the health record, precertification/prior authorization request form, copy of the health insurance ID card, and a pen. For the electronic method, access the Simulation Playground in SCMO.	20		
2. Using the health record, determine the service or procedure that requires precertification/preauthorization.	20*		

3.	For the paper method, complete the Precertification/Prior Authorization Request form. For the electronic method, click on the Form Repository icon in SCMO. Select Prior Authorization Request from the left INFO PANEL. Use the Patient Search button at the bottom to find the patient. Complete the remaining fields of the form.	20		
4.	Proofread the completed form and make any revisions needed.	20		
5.	Paper method: File the document in the health record after it is faxed to the insurance carrier. Electronic method: Print and fax or electronically send the form to the insurance company and save the form to the patient's record.	20		
	Total Points	100		

Comments

CAAHEP Competencies	Step(s)
VIII.P.2 Verify eligibility for services including documentation	Entire procedure
VIII.P.3. Obtain precertification or preauthorization including documentation	Entire procedure
ABHES Competencies	**Step(s)**
7. Administrative Procedures c. Perform billing and collection procedures	Entire procedure

Procedure 18.4   Complete an Insurance Claim Form

Name _____ Date _____ Score _____

Task: To accurately complete a CMS-1500 Health Insurance Claim Form.

Equipment and Supplies:
- Patient's health record
- Copy of patient's insurance ID card or cards
- Patient registration/intake form
- Encounter form
- Insurance claims processing guidelines (Table 18.2)
- Blank CMS-1500 Health Insurance Claim Form (Work Product 18.1)

Background: Almost all medical billing is done electronically through practice management billing software. The paper CMS-1500 Health Insurance Claim Form is provided only to help students practice and develop their medical billing skills.

Directions: Complete each block (as appropriate) of the CMS-1500 (see Table 18.2 for block descriptions).

Scenario: Mr. Walter Biller had an appointment with Dr. Walden on November 16, 20XX. He came in for an influenza vaccine, and while he was there, he wanted Dr. Walden to look at his ear because he was having problems hearing. His right ear canal was impacted with cerumen, which was irrigated and the cerumen was removed during the visit.

Patient Demographics	Clinic and Provider Information	
Walter B. Biller (patient and insured)	Walden-Martin Family Medical Clinic	
87 Willoughby Lane	1234 Anystreet	
Anytown, AL 12345-1234	Anytown, AL 12345	
Phone: 123-237-3748	123-123-1234	
DOB: 01/04/1970	POS – 04 Independent clinic	
SSN: 285-77-7796	Established patient of Julie Walden, MD	
HIPAA form on file: Yes – March 19, 20XX	Federal Tax ID# 651249831	
Signature on file: Yes – March 19, 20XX	NPI# 1467253823	
Insurance Information		
Account Number: 16611		
Aetna		
Policy/ID Number: CH8327753		
Group Number: 33347H		
Diagnosis:	**ICD-10-CM code**	
Impacted cerumen, right ear	H61.21	
Service	**CPT Code**	**Fee**
Est. minimal OV	99211	$24.00
Cerumen removal	69210	$46.00
Vaccine – Flu, 3 Y+	90658	$24.00
Preventive - Flu Administration	G0008	$7.00

Standard: Complete the procedure and all critical steps in _____ minutes with a minimum score of 85% within two attempts (*or as indicated by the instructor*).

Scoring: Divide the points earned by the total possible points. Failure to perform a critical step, indicated by an asterisk (*), results in grade no higher than an 84% (*or as indicated by the instructor*).

Time: Began_____ Ended_____ Total minutes: _____

Steps:	Point Value	Attempt 1	Attempt 2
1. Gather the documents required to complete the claim form.	10		
2. Complete the claim form using a pen. Use capital letters. Do not use punctuation (commas or dollar signs) unless indicated in the insurance manual or guidelines. Use a hyphen to hyphenate last names.	10		
3. Using the patient's health insurance ID card, determine the type of insurance, and the insurance ID number. Enter this information into block 1 and 1a.	10		
4. Using the ID card, the encounter form, and the registration/intake form, determine the patient's information and insured individual's information. Accurately complete blocks 2, 3, 5, 6, 9, and 10 a-c by entering in the patient's information. Complete 4, 7, and 11, a-d with the insured's information.	10		
5. Complete blocks 12 and 13 by entering "signature on file" and the date.	10		
6. Accurately enter the physician or supplier information by completing blocks 14 through 23. Use the eight (8)–digit format (MM/DD/YYYY) when needed.	10		
7. Using the encounter form, complete the appropriate blocks from 24A through 24H. **Note**: • Block 24A: Enter the dates of service, both From and To. For ambulatory services, enter the same date in the FROM and TO fields. Enter a date for each procedure, service, or supply in eight (8)–digit format (MM/DD/YYYY). • Block 24F: Enter the charge for the listed service or procedure. *Do not use commas when reporting dollar amounts.* The cents column is the small column to the right. • Block 24G: Enter the number of days or units. This block is usually used for multiple visits, units of supplies, anesthesia units or minutes, or oxygen volume. If only one service is performed, enter 1.0	10		
8. Complete blocks 24I through 27 by entering information on the provider's or healthcare facility where the service was provided and the patient's account number. Check the correct box to indicate acceptance of assignment of benefits.	10		
9. Complete blocks 28 through 29 by entering the total charges, total amount paid, and the total amount due. Complete blocks 31 through 33a by entering in the provider's and facility's information.	10		
10. Review the claim for accuracy and completeness before submitting. Correct any errors or missing information.	10*		
Total Points	100		

Comments

CAAHEP Competencies	Step(s)
VIII.P.4. Complete an insurance claim form	Entire procedure
ABHES Competencies	**Step(s)**
7. Administrative Procedures d. Process insurance claims	Entire procedure

Work Product 18.1 CMS-1500 Health Insurance Claim Form

HEALTH INSURANCE CLAIM FORM

APPROVED BY NATIONAL UNIFORM CLAIM COMMITTEE (NUCC) 02/12

CARRIER

PICA							PICA	

1. MEDICARE ☐ (Medicare#) MEDICAID ☐ (Medicaid#) TRICARE ☐ (ID#/DoD#) CHAMPVA ☐ (Member ID#) GROUP HEALTH PLAN ☐ (ID#) FECA BLK LUNG ☐ (ID#) OTHER ☐ (ID#) **1a.** INSURED'S I.D. NUMBER (For Program in Item 1)

2. PATIENT'S NAME (Last Name, First Name, Middle Initial)

3. PATIENT'S BIRTH DATE MM DD YY SEX M ☐ F ☐

4. INSURED'S NAME (Last Name, First Name, Middle Initial)

5. PATIENT'S ADDRESS (No., Street)

6. PATIENT RELATIONSHIP TO INSURED Self ☐ Spouse ☐ Child ☐ Other ☐

7. INSURED'S ADDRESS (No., Street)

CITY STATE

8. RESERVED FOR NUCC USE

CITY STATE

ZIP CODE TELEPHONE (Include Area Code) ( )

ZIP CODE TELEPHONE (Include Area Code) ( )

9. OTHER INSURED'S NAME (Last Name, First Name, Middle Initial)

10. IS PATIENT'S CONDITION RELATED TO:

11. INSURED'S POLICY GROUP OR FECA NUMBER

a. OTHER INSURED'S POLICY OR GROUP NUMBER

a. EMPLOYMENT? (Current or Previous) YES ☐ NO ☐

a. INSURED'S DATE OF BIRTH MM DD YY SEX M ☐ F ☐

b. RESERVED FOR NUCC USE

b. AUTO ACCIDENT? YES ☐ NO ☐ PLACE (State)

b. OTHER CLAIM ID (Designated by NUCC)

c. RESERVED FOR NUCC USE

c. OTHER ACCIDENT? YES ☐ NO ☐

c. INSURANCE PLAN NAME OR PROGRAM NAME

d. INSURANCE PLAN NAME OR PROGRAM NAME

10d. CLAIM CODES (Designated by NUCC)

d. IS THERE ANOTHER HEALTH BENEFIT PLAN? YES ☐ NO ☐ If yes, complete items 9, 9a, and 9d.

READ BACK OF FORM BEFORE COMPLETING & SIGNING THIS FORM.
12. PATIENT'S OR AUTHORIZED PERSON'S SIGNATURE I authorize the release of any medical or other information necessary to process this claim. I also request payment of government benefits either to myself or to the party who accepts assignment below.

SIGNED _____ DATE _____

13. INSURED'S OR AUTHORIZED PERSON'S SIGNATURE I authorize payment of medical benefits to the undersigned physician or supplier for services described below.

SIGNED _____

PATIENT AND INSURED INFORMATION

14. DATE OF CURRENT ILLNESS, INJURY, or PREGNANCY (LMP) MM DD YY QUAL.

15. OTHER DATE QUAL. MM DD YY

16. DATES PATIENT UNABLE TO WORK IN CURRENT OCCUPATION FROM MM DD YY TO MM DD YY

17. NAME OF REFERRING PROVIDER OR OTHER SOURCE

17a. 17b. NPI

18. HOSPITALIZATION DATES RELATED TO CURRENT SERVICES FROM MM DD YY TO MM DD YY

19. ADDITIONAL CLAIM INFORMATION (Designated by NUCC)

20. OUTSIDE LAB? YES ☐ NO ☐ $ CHARGES

21. DIAGNOSIS OR NATURE OF ILLNESS OR INJURY Relate A-L to service line below (24E) ICD Ind.

A. ___ B. ___ C. ___ D. ___
E. ___ F. ___ G. ___ H. ___
I. ___ J. ___ K. ___ L. ___

22. RESUBMISSION CODE ORIGINAL REF. NO.

23. PRIOR AUTHORIZATION NUMBER

24. A. DATE(S) OF SERVICE						B. PLACE OF SERVICE	C. EMG	D. PROCEDURES, SERVICES, OR SUPPLIES (Explain Unusual Circumstances) CPT/HCPCS | MODIFIER	E. DIAGNOSIS POINTER	F. $ CHARGES	G. DAYS OR UNITS	H. EPSDT Family Plan	I. ID. QUAL.	J. RENDERING PROVIDER ID. #
From			To											
MM	DD	YY	MM	DD	YY									
1													NPI	
2													NPI	
3													NPI	
4													NPI	
5													NPI	
6													NPI	

25. FEDERAL TAX I.D. NUMBER SSN ☐ EIN ☐

26. PATIENT'S ACCOUNT NO.

27. ACCEPT ASSIGNMENT? (For govt. claims, see back) YES ☐ NO ☐

28. TOTAL CHARGE $

29. AMOUNT PAID $

30. Rsvd for NUCC Use

31. SIGNATURE OF PHYSICIAN OR SUPPLIER INCLUDING DEGREES OR CREDENTIALS (I certify that the statements on the reverse apply to this bill and are made a part thereof.)

SIGNED _____ DATE _____

32. SERVICE FACILITY LOCATION INFORMATION

a. NPI b.

33. BILLING PROVIDER INFO & PH # ( )

a. NPI b.

PHYSICIAN OR SUPPLIER INFORMATION

NUCC Instruction Manual available at: www.nucc.org **PLEASE PRINT OR TYPE** APPROVED OMB-0938-1197 FORM 1500 (02-12)

Procedure 18.5   Utilize Medical Necessity Guidelines: Respond to a "Medical Necessity Denied" Claim

Name _____   Date _____   Score _____

Task: To resolve the insurance company's denial of a claim for medical necessity by completing an accurate claim.

Equipment and Supplies:
- Paper method: Patient's health record, copy of patient's insurance ID card or cards, patient registration form, encounter form, blank CMS-1500 Health Insurance Claim Form (Work Product 18.2), and a pen
- Electronic method: SimChart for the Medical Office
- Insurance denial letter or scenario (see below)

Scenario: You are working at Walden-Martin Family Medical Clinic, 1234 Anystreet, Anytown, AL 12345 (phone: 123-123-1234). You receive a letter indicating that Medicare has denied the following claim for not being medically necessary:

Patient: Norma B. Washington	DOB: 08/07/1944	Policy/ID Number: 847744144A
Date of Service: 06/13/20XX	ICD: G43.101 (Migraine)	CPT: J3420 (B-12 injection)
Provider: Julie Walden MD		

You did some research and the information above was the only information sent to Medicare for that encounter. The following information was the correct information for the encounter:

Patient: Norma B. Washington	DOB: 08/01/1944	Date of Service: 06/15/20XX
ICD: G43.101 (Migraine)	CPT: J1885 (Toradol 15 mg—$15.50) and 90772 (Injection, Ther/Proph/Diag—$25.00)	
ICD: D51.0 (Vitamin B$_{12}$ deficiency anemia) CPT: J3420 (B$_{12}$ injection—$24.00) and 90772 (Injection, Ther/Proph/Diag—$25.00)		
To be billed to: Medicare, 1234 Insurance Road, Anytown, AL 12345-1234		

Standard: Complete the procedure and all critical steps in _____ minutes with a minimum score of 85% within two attempts (*or as indicated by the instructor*).

Scoring: Divide the points earned by the total possible points. Failure to perform a critical step, indicated by an asterisk (*), results in grade no higher than an 84% (*or as indicated by the instructor*).

Time: Began_____ Ended_____ Total minutes: _____

Steps:	Point Value	Attempt 1	Attempt 2
1. Review the insurance denial letter (scenario) carefully. Compare the patient's information from the denial letter to the health record, claim, and encounter form. Look for errors in the patient's name and date of birth.	20*		
2. Compare the insurance denial letter (scenario) to the health record, claim, and encounter form. Look for errors in the date of service, the diagnosis, and the procedure codes. The procedure must be medically necessary for the diagnosis indicated.	20*		

3.	Complete a claim (either CMS-1500 or an electronic claim using SimChart) by entering in the information about the carrier, patient, and insured.	20		
4.	Enter the information regarding the physician, procedures, and diagnosis. Make sure to include all of the information from the encounter.	20		
5.	Proofread the claim form for accuracy before submitting the claim.	20		
	Total Points	100		

Comments

CAAHEP Competencies	Step(s)
IX.P.3. Utilize medical necessity guidelines	Entire procedure
ABHES Competencies	**Step(s)**
7. Administrative Procedures c. Perform billing and collection procedures	Entire procedure

Work Product 18.2 CMS-1500 Health Insurance Claim Form

HEALTH INSURANCE CLAIM FORM

APPROVED BY NATIONAL UNIFORM CLAIM COMMITTEE (NUCC) 02/12

| | PICA | | | | | | | | PICA | |

1. MEDICARE ☐ (Medicare#) MEDICAID ☐ (Medicaid#) TRICARE ☐ (ID#/DoD#) CHAMPVA ☐ (Member ID#) GROUP HEALTH PLAN ☐ (ID#) FECA BLK LUNG ☐ (ID#) OTHER ☐ (ID#) **1a. INSURED'S I.D. NUMBER** (For Program in Item 1)

2. PATIENT'S NAME (Last Name, First Name, Middle Initial)

3. PATIENT'S BIRTH DATE MM | DD | YY   SEX M ☐ F ☐

4. INSURED'S NAME (Last Name, First Name, Middle Initial)

5. PATIENT'S ADDRESS (No., Street)

6. PATIENT RELATIONSHIP TO INSURED Self ☐ Spouse ☐ Child ☐ Other ☐

7. INSURED'S ADDRESS (No., Street)

CITY | STATE

8. RESERVED FOR NUCC USE

CITY | STATE

ZIP CODE | TELEPHONE (Include Area Code) ( )

ZIP CODE | TELEPHONE (Include Area Code) ( )

9. OTHER INSURED'S NAME (Last Name, First Name, Middle Initial)

10. IS PATIENT'S CONDITION RELATED TO:

11. INSURED'S POLICY GROUP OR FECA NUMBER

a. OTHER INSURED'S POLICY OR GROUP NUMBER

a. EMPLOYMENT? (Current or Previous) ☐ YES ☐ NO

a. INSURED'S DATE OF BIRTH MM | DD | YY   SEX M ☐ F ☐

b. RESERVED FOR NUCC USE

b. AUTO ACCIDENT? ☐ YES ☐ NO   PLACE (State)

b. OTHER CLAIM ID (Designated by NUCC)

c. RESERVED FOR NUCC USE

c. OTHER ACCIDENT? ☐ YES ☐ NO

c. INSURANCE PLAN NAME OR PROGRAM NAME

d. INSURANCE PLAN NAME OR PROGRAM NAME

10d. CLAIM CODES (Designated by NUCC)

d. IS THERE ANOTHER HEALTH BENEFIT PLAN? ☐ YES ☐ NO *If yes*, complete items 9, 9a, and 9d.

READ BACK OF FORM BEFORE COMPLETING & SIGNING THIS FORM.
12. PATIENT'S OR AUTHORIZED PERSON'S SIGNATURE I authorize the release of any medical or other information necessary to process this claim. I also request payment of government benefits either to myself or to the party who accepts assignment below.

SIGNED _____ DATE _____

13. INSURED'S OR AUTHORIZED PERSON'S SIGNATURE I authorize payment of medical benefits to the undersigned physician or supplier for services described below.

SIGNED _____

14. DATE OF CURRENT ILLNESS, INJURY, or PREGNANCY (LMP) MM | DD | YY   QUAL.

15. OTHER DATE QUAL. | MM | DD | YY

16. DATES PATIENT UNABLE TO WORK IN CURRENT OCCUPATION FROM MM | DD | YY TO MM | DD | YY

17. NAME OF REFERRING PROVIDER OR OTHER SOURCE
17a.
17b. NPI

18. HOSPITALIZATION DATES RELATED TO CURRENT SERVICES FROM MM | DD | YY TO MM | DD | YY

19. ADDITIONAL CLAIM INFORMATION (Designated by NUCC)

20. OUTSIDE LAB? ☐ YES ☐ NO $ CHARGES

21. DIAGNOSIS OR NATURE OF ILLNESS OR INJURY Relate A-L to service line below (24E)   ICD Ind.

A. |____ B. |____ C. |____ D. |____
E. |____ F. |____ G. |____ H. |____
I. |____ J. |____ K. |____ L. |____

22. RESUBMISSION CODE | ORIGINAL REF. NO.

23. PRIOR AUTHORIZATION NUMBER

24. A. DATE(S) OF SERVICE						B. PLACE OF SERVICE	C. EMG	D. PROCEDURES, SERVICES, OR SUPPLIES (Explain Unusual Circumstances) CPT/HCPCS | MODIFIER	E. DIAGNOSIS POINTER	F. $ CHARGES	G. DAYS OR UNITS	H. EPSDT Family Plan	I. ID. QUAL.	J. RENDERING PROVIDER ID. #
	From MM DD YY			To MM DD YY										
1														NPI
2														NPI
3														NPI
4														NPI
5														NPI
6														NPI

25. FEDERAL TAX I.D. NUMBER ☐ SSN ☐ EIN

26. PATIENT'S ACCOUNT NO.

27. ACCEPT ASSIGNMENT? (For govt. claims, see back) ☐ YES ☐ NO

28. TOTAL CHARGE $

29. AMOUNT PAID $

30. Rsvd for NUCC Use

31. SIGNATURE OF PHYSICIAN OR SUPPLIER INCLUDING DEGREES OR CREDENTIALS (I certify that the statements on the reverse apply to this bill and are made a part thereof.)

SIGNED _____ DATE _____

32. SERVICE FACILITY LOCATION INFORMATION
a. NPI b.

33. BILLING PROVIDER INFO & PH # ( )
a. NPI b.

NUCC Instruction Manual available at: www.nucc.org   **PLEASE PRINT OR TYPE**   APPROVED OMB-0938-1197 FORM 1500 (02-12)

CARRIER *PATIENT AND INSURED INFORMATION* *PHYSICIAN OR SUPPLIER INFORMATION*

Procedure 18.6   Inform a Patient of Financial Obligations for Services Rendered

Name _____ Date _____ Score _____

Tasks: Inform patient of his/her financial obligation and to demonstrate professionalism and sensitivity when discussing the patient's billing record.

Equipment and Supplies:
- Facility's payment policy
- Copy of patient's insurance card (or see information in the scenario)
- Patient's account record (or see information in the scenario)

Obtaining Payments – WMFM Clinic Policy
- For patients with copayments, all copayments must be collected before the patient leaves the clinic.
- For patients with balances overdue:
  - Patients must pay 20% of the balance before an appointment can be scheduled.
  - Or patients can establish a 6- or 12-month interest-free payment plan, making the first payment before the next visit can be scheduled.
- Payments can be made using VISA, Mastercard, personal check (no starter checks accepted), or cash. Payments can also be made online.

Scenario #1: Mr. Walter Biller arrives for his appointment. You need to check his eligibility for services and also if he has a copayment for today's visit. His insurance information: account number: 16611; Aetna, Policy/ID Number: CH8327753; and Group Number: 33347H

Scenario #2: Christi Brown is meeting with you regarding the bill she received in the mail. She called to make the appointment and she voiced her confusion about the bill. She stated that she thought her insurance covered everything. You check her record and see that she met her deductible and now needs to pay 20% of the billed amount. She owes $170.

Directions: Role-play the scenarios with a peer. The peer will be the insurance representative in Scenario #1, and then the patient in Scenario #2. You will be the medical assistant. You need to be professional and sensitive when working with patients regarding payments. You also need to follow the clinic's policy.

Standard: Complete the procedure and all critical steps in _____ minutes with a minimum score of 85% within two attempts (*or as indicated by the instructor*).

Scoring: Divide the points earned by the total possible points. Failure to perform a critical step, indicated by an asterisk (*), results in grade no higher than an 84% (*or as indicated by the instructor*).

Time: Began_____ Ended_____ Total minutes: _____

Steps:	Point Value	Attempt 1	Attempt 2
Scenario #1: Role-play with a peer who will be the insurance representative. 1. Contact the patient's insurance company and verify the patient's eligibility for services. Provide the representative with the patient's information. Find out if the patient has a copayment for today's visit. Document the information obtained.	20*		

Comments

CAAHEP Competencies	Step(s)
VII.A.1. Demonstrate professionalism when discussing patient's billing record	4, 7
VII.A.2. Display sensitivity when requesting payment for services rendered	4, 7
VIII.P.2. Verify eligibility for services including documentation	1
VII.P.4. Inform a patient of financial obligations for services rendered	2, 5
ABHES Competencies	**Step(s)**
7. Administrative Procedures c. Perform billing and collection procedures	Entire procedure

Patient Accounts and Practice Management

CAAHEP Competencies	Assessment
II.C.1. Demonstrate knowledge of basic math computations	Skills and Concepts – D. 13
VII.C.1.a. Define the following bookkeeping terms: charges	Skills and Concepts – B. 2.4
VII.C.1.b. Define the following bookkeeping terms: payments	Skills and Concepts – B. 2.5
VII.C.1.c. Define the following bookkeeping terms: accounts receivable	Skills and Concepts – B. 2.2
VII.C.1.d. Define the following bookkeeping terms: accounts payable	Skills and Concepts – B. 2.1
VII.C.1.e. Define the following bookkeeping terms: adjustments	Skills and Concepts – B. 2.3
VII.C.2. Describe banking procedures as related to the ambulatory care setting	Skills and Concepts – D. 1-5
VII.C.3.a. Identify precautions for accepting the following types of payments: cash	Skills and Concepts – D. 7
VII.C.3.b. Identify precautions for accepting the following types of payments: check	Skills and Concepts – D. 6
VII.C.3.c. Identify precautions for accepting the following types of payments: credit card	Skills and Concepts – D. 8
VII.C.3.d. Identify precautions for accepting the following types of payments: debit card	Skills and Concepts – D. 8
VII.C.4.a. Describe types of adjustments made to patient accounts including: non-sufficient funds (NSF) check	Skills and Concepts – C. 6
VII.C.4.b. Describe types of adjustments made to patient accounts including: collection agency transaction	Skills and Concepts – C. 4
VII.C.4.c. Describe types of adjustments made to patient accounts including: credit balance	Skills and Concepts – C. 5
VII.C.4.d. Describe types of adjustments made to patient accounts including: third party	Skills and Concepts – C. 3

CAAHEP Competencies	Assessment
VII.C.5. Identify types of information contained in the patient's billing record	Skills and Concepts – C. 7
VII.C.6. Explain patient financial obligations for services rendered	Workplace Applications – 1
VII.P.1.a. Perform accounts receivable procedures to patient accounts including posting: charges	Procedure 19.1
VII.P.1.b. Perform accounts receivable procedures to patient accounts including posting: payments	Procedure 19.1, 19.3
VII.P.1.c. Perform accounts receivable procedures to patient accounts including posting: adjustments	Procedure 19.3
VII.P.2. Prepare a bank deposit	Procedure 19.4
VII.P.3. Obtain accurate patient billing information	Procedure 19.2
VII.P.4. Inform a patient of financial obligations for services rendered	Procedure 19.2
VII.A.1. Demonstrate professionalism when discussing patient's billing record	Procedure 19.2
VII.A.2. Display sensitivity when requesting payment for services rendered	Procedure 19.2
ABHES Competencies	**Assessment**
1. General Orientation d. List the general responsibilities and skills of the medical assistant	Skills and Concepts – D.
7. Administrative Procedures c. Perform billing and collection procedures	Procedures 19.1, 19.2, 19.3, 19.4

VOCABULARY REVIEW

Using the word pool on the right, find the correct word to match the definition. Write the word on the line after the definition.

Group A

1. The person legally responsible for the entire bill

   _____

2. A document sent by the insurance company to the provider and the patient explaining the allowed charge amount, the amount reimbursed for services, and the patient's financial responsibilities

   _____

3. The process of recording financial transactions

   _____

4. A manual bookkeeping system that uses a day sheet to record all financial transactions for the date of service and maintains patient account balances by using physical ledger cards

   _____

5. Poor, needy, impoverished _____

6. To come into or acquire _____

7. A list of fixed fees for services _____

8. A minor who has been granted emancipation by the court; the minor can assume the rights and responsibilities of adulthood

   _____

9. The amount of money the healthcare facility has in the bank that can be withdrawn as cash _____

10. A running balance of all financial transactions for a specific patient

    _____

Word Pool
- bookkeeping
- incurred
- cash on hand
- patient account
- guarantor
- pegboard system
- fee schedule
- explanation of benefits
- emancipated minor
- indigent

Group B

1. Something of value that cannot be touched physically

   _____

2. Hostile and aggressive _____

3. A special court established to handle small claims or debts, without the services of lawyers _____

4. A chronologic file used as a reminder that something must be dealt with on a certain date _____

5. All property available for the payment of debts

   _____

6. An oath or swear word _____

7. An individual or party who brings the suit to court

   _____

8. Debt that is not guaranteed by something of value; credit card debt is the most common type _____

9. An individual assigned to make financial decisions about the estate of a deceased patient _____

10. The coordinator of financial resources assigned by the court during a bankruptcy case _____

Word Pool
- belligerent
- expletive
- tickler file
- intangible
- executor
- assets
- unsecured debt
- trustee
- small claims court
- plaintiff

Group C

1. Money the bank pays the account holder on the amount in their account for using the money in the account

   _____

2. Global technology that includes imbedded microchips that store and protect cardholder data; also called *chip and PIN* and *chip and signature* _____

3. Money in a bank account that is not assigned to pay for any office expenses _____

4. An imitation intended to be passed off fraudulently or deceptively as genuine; forgery _____

5. A fixed compensation periodically paid to a person for regular work _____

6. The central bank of the United States _____

7. The misuse of a healthcare facility's funds for personal gain

   _____

8. An individual or business against whom a lawsuit is filed

   _____

9. To bring into agreement _____

10. A document guaranteeing payment of a specific amount of money to the payer named on the document _____

Word Pool
- defendant
- interest
- Federal Reserve Bank
- discretionary income
- negotiable instrument
- counterfeit
- EMV chip technology
- embezzlement
- reconciliation
- salaried

ABBREVIATIONS

Write out what each of the following abbreviations stands for.

1. EOB _____

2. A/R _____

3. A/P _____

4. TILA _____

5. FTC _____

6. PIN _____

7. POS _____

8. EFT _____

SKILLS AND CONCEPTS

Answer the following questions. Write your answer on the line or in the space provided.

A. Managing Funds in the Healthcare Facility

1. What items should appear on the financial records of any business at all times? _____

   _____

   _____

   _____

   _____

B. Bookkeeping in the Healthcare Facility

1. Examine the fee schedule and answer the following questions.

FEE SCHEDULE

BLACKBURN PRIMARY CARE ASSOCIATES, PC
1990 Turquiose Drive
Blackburn, WI 54937
608-459-8857

| **Federal Tax ID Number:** | 00-0000000 | **BCBS Group Number: 14982** |
| | | **Medicare Group Number: 14982** |

OFFICE VISIT, NEW PATIENT

Focused, 99201	$45.00
Expanded, 99202	$55.00
Intermediate, 99203	$60.00
Extended, 99204	$95.00
Comprehensive, 99205	$195.00
Consultation, 99245	$250.00

OFFICE VISIT, ESTABLISHED PATIENT

Minimal, 99211	$40.00
Focused, 99212	$48.00
Intermediate, 99213	$55.00
Extended, 99214	$65.00
Comprehensive, 99215	$195.00

OFFICE PROCEDURES

ECG, 12 lead, 93000	$55.00
Stress ECG, Treadmill, 93015	$295.00
Sigmoidoscopy, Flex; 45330	$145.00
Spirometry, 94010	$50.00
Cerumen Removal, 69210	$40.00
Collection & Handling	
Lab Specimen, 99000	$9.00
Venipuncture, 35415	$9.00
Urinalysis, 81000	$20.00
Urinalysis, 81002 (Dip Only)	$12.00
Influenza Injection, 90724	$20.00
Pneumococcal Injection, 90732	$20.00
Oral Polio, 90712	$15.00
DTaP, 90700	$20.00
Tetanus Toxoid, 90703	$15.00
MMR, 90707	$25.00
HIB, 90737	$20.00
Hepatitis B, newborn to age 11 years, 90744	$60.00
Hepatitis B, 11-19 years, 90745	$60.00
Hepatitis B, 20 years and above 90746	$60.00
Intramuscular Injection, 90788	
Penicillin	$30.00
Cephtriaxone	$25.00
Solu-Medrol	$23.00
Vitamin B-12	$13.00
Subcutaneous Injection, 90782	
Epinephrine	$18.00
Susphrine	$25.00
Insulin, U-100	$15.00

COMMON DIAGNOSTIC CODES

Acute coronary thrombosis without myocardial infarction I24.0
Other forms of acute ischemic heart disease I24.8
Chronic ischemic heart disease I25.9
Essential hypertension (arterial)(benign) (essential)(malignant)(primary)(systemic) I10
Hypertensive heart disease with heart failure I11.0
Unspecified asthma, uncomplicated J45.909
Asthma with COPD J44.9
Other asthma J45.998
Unspecified asthma with status asthmaticus J45.902
Postural kyphosis M40.00
Osteoporosis M81.0
Acute otitis media H66.0
Chronic otittis media H66.3

a. What is the charge for a consultation? _____

b. What is the charge for CPT code 99203? _____

c. What is the most expensive procedure on the list? _____

d. Which injection is more expensive, insulin or vitamin B_{12}? _____

2. Match the following terms with the correct definition:

Terms	**Definitions**
1. Accounts payable _____	a. Money that is expected but has not yet been received
2. Accounts receivable _____	b. Fees applied to the patient account when services are rendered
3. Adjustments _____	c. The management of debt incurred and not yet paid
4. Charges _____	d. Money given to the provider in exchange for services
5. Payments _____	e. Credits posted to the patient account when the provider's fee exceeds the amount allowed stated on the EOB

C. Accounts Receivable

1. What are the pitfalls of fee adjustments? _____

_____

_____

_____

_____

2. Briefly explain how "skips" can be traced. _____

_____

_____

_____

_____

_____

3. When a provider's fee exceeds the allowed amount stated on the explanation of benefits from the insurance company, a(n) _____ is posted to the patient account record for that difference.

4. When a patient account is turned over to a collection agency, what adjustment is posted to the account?

_____

_____

5. When a patient has a credit balance on his or her account, what adjustment is posted to the account?

_____

_____

_____

6. Describe the adjustments that are made to the patient's account when an NSF check is received by the healthcare facility.

_____

_____

_____

_____

7. What information should be included on the patient ledger? _____

_____

_____

_____

_____

_____

D. Accounts Payable

1. In the ambulatory care setting, what is the checking account used for? _____

_____

_____

2. In the ambulatory care setting, what is a savings account used for? _____

_____

_____

3. You are a medical assistant in a small practice and have been told that you now have the responsibility for paying the bills by writing out and signing the checks. What is the first action you need to take before writing out the first check?

_____

_____

4. Name six activities that can be done with basic online banking services.

a. _____

b. _____

c. _____

d. _____

e. _____

f. _____

5. List the four requirements for a check to be negotiable.

    a. _____

    b. _____

    c. _____

    d. _____

6. Describe five precautions for accepting checks in the healthcare facility.

    a. _____

    b. _____

    c. _____

    d. _____

    e. _____

7. Describe four precautions to take if a patient is paying with cash.

    a. _____

    b. _____

    c. _____

    d. _____

8. Describe precautions to take when a patient pays with a debit card or a credit card. _____

_____

_____

_____

_____

_____

9. Describe the banking procedures as related to the ambulatory care setting and include the medical assistant's role with each procedure.

    a. Making bank deposits: _____

_____

_____

_____

    b. Preparing a bank deposit:_____

        _____

        _____

        _____

    c. Endorsing checks: _____

        _____

        _____

        _____

    d. Writing checks:_____

        _____

        _____

        _____

10. Describe three ways to do a mobile deposit of a check.

    a.   _____

    b.   _____

    c.   _____

11. Describe each type of endorsement.

    a. Blank endorsement:_____

        _____

        _____

        _____

    b. Restrictive endorsement: _____

        _____

        _____

        _____

    c. Special endorsement: _____

        _____

        _____

        _____

INTERNET ACTIVITIES

1. Using online resources, research the role of an accountant. Create a poster presentation, a PowerPoint presentation, or write a paper summarizing your research. Include the following points in your project:
   a. Why most healthcare providers employ one to handle financials for the office
   b. What an accountant does for the provider
   c. How a medical assistant helps the accountant do his or her job

2. Using online resources, research mobile deposit technology. Create a poster presentation, a PowerPoint presentation, or write a paper summarizing your research. Include the following points in your project:
   a. Describe three different mobile deposit technologies available for healthcare facilities.
   b. Describe which technology would work best for a small provider's office, large provider's office, and physical therapy rehabilitation facility.

Procedure 19.1 Post Charges and Payments to Patient Accounts

Name _____ Date _____ Score _____

Task: To enter charges into the patient account record manually and electronically.

Equipment and Supplies:
- Patient account ledger card (Work Product 19.1)
- SimChart for the Medical Office software
- Encounter form/superbill
- Provider's fee schedule

Scenario: Ken Thomas is a returning patient of Dr. Martin. He makes his $50 copayment at the time of the office visit.

Standard: Complete the procedure and all critical steps in _____ minutes with a minimum score of 85% within two attempts (*or as indicated by the instructor*).

Scoring: Divide the points earned by the total possible points. Failure to perform a critical step, indicated by an asterisk (*), results in grade no higher than an 84% (*or as indicated by the instructor*).

Time: Began_____ Ended_____ Total minutes: _____

Steps for Posting Charges Manually:	Point Value	Attempt 1	Attempt 2
1. For new patients, create the patient account by entering the following information on a patient account ledger card: • Patient's full name, address, and at least two contact phone numbers • Date of birth • Health insurance information, including the subscriber number, group number, and effective date • Subscriber's name and date of birth (if the subscriber is not the patient) For returning patients, review the account record to see whether a balance is due. If there is a balance, bring this to the patient's attention when he or she comes for the appointment. Respectfully explain that the provider would appreciate a payment on the previous balance before he or she can care for the patient.	50		
2. After seeing the patient, the provider completes the encounter form, which includes all procedures and the associated fee schedule. Using the completed encounter form (see Figure 19.1 in textbook), enter the charges manually on the ledger card for the patient's account record. Total all the charges on the encounter form for the services rendered. Then subtract the copayment made from the total charges. The previous balance, if any, is added to this new total. Use the following worksheet to calculate the new balance. The new balance due amount should be presented to the patient before he or she leaves the healthcare facility. | Total Charges	$ | | Amount paid (copayment) | $ | | + Previous balance (if any) | $ | | = New Balance Due | $ |	50*		
Total Points	100		

Steps for Posting Charges in SimChart for the Medical Office			
1. After logging into SimChart, locate the established patient by clicking on Find Patient, enter the patient's name, verify DOB, and click on the radio button. This will bring you to the Clinical Care tab. If there is no encounter shown, create an encounter by clicking on Office Visit under Info Panel on the left, select a visit type, and click on Save. Once an encounter has been created, return to the Patient Dashboard and click on the Superbill link on the right (or click on the Coding and Billing tab).	20		
2. From the Superbill area, in the Encounters Not Coded section, click on the encounter (in blue). On page 1, enter the diagnosis in the Diagnosis field and document the services provided (additional services are found on pages 2-3 of the Superbill).	20		
3. Complete the information needed on page 4 of the Superbill and submit.	20*		
4. Click on Ledger on the left and search for your patient. Once your patient has been located, click on the arrow across from the name in the ledger.	20		
5. Enter the payment received. The balance will be auto-calculated for you.	20		
Total Points	100		

Comments

CAAHEP Competencies	Step(s)
VII.P.1.a. Perform accounts receivable procedures to patient accounts including posting: charges	Manual: 2 SimChart: 2
VII.P.1.b. Perform accounts receivable procedures to patient accounts including posting: payments	Manual: 2 SimChart: 5
ABHES Competencies	**Step(s)**
7. Administrative Procedures c. Perform billing and collection procedures	Entire procedure

Work Product 19.1 Ledger

Ledger:

Blue Cross Blue Shield
ID # KT4496785
Group # 55124T
Subscriber: Ken Thomas   Ken Thomas
398 Larkin Avenue
DOB: 10/25/1961   Anytown, Anystate 12345-1234

Date	Service Description	Charges	Payments	Adjustments	Balance

Procedure 19.2 Inform a Patient of Financial Obligations for Services Rendered

Name _____ **Date** _____ **Score** _____

Tasks: Inform a patient of his/her financial obligation and demonstrate professionalism and sensitivity when discussing the patient's billing record.

Equipment and Supplies:
- Facility's payment policy
- Copy of patient's insurance card (or see information in the scenario)
- Patient's account record (or see information in the scenario)

Obtaining Payments – WMFM Clinic Policy

- For patients with copayments, all copayments must be collected before the patient leaves the clinic.
- For patients with balances overdue:
  - Patients must pay 20% of the balance before an appointment can be scheduled.
  - Or patients can establish a 6- or 12-month interest-free payment plan, making the first payment before the next visit can be scheduled.
- Payments can be made using VISA, Mastercard, personal check (no starter checks accepted), or cash. Payments can also be made online.

Scenario #1: Mr. Walter Biller arrives for his appointment. You need to check his eligibility for services and also if he has a copayment for today's visit. His insurance information: account number: 16611; Aetna, Policy/ID Number: CH8327753; and Group Number: 33347H

Scenario #2: Christi Brown is meeting with you regarding the bill she received in the mail. She called to make the appointment and she voiced her confusion about the bill. She stated that she thought her insurance covered everything. You check her record and see that she met her deductible and now needs to pay 20% of the billed amount. She owes $170.

Directions: Role-play the scenarios with a peer. The peer will be the insurance representative in Scenario #1, and then the patient in Scenario #2. You will be the medical assistant. You need to be professional and sensitive when working with patients regarding payments. You also need to follow the clinic's policy.

Standard: Complete the procedure and all critical steps in _____ minutes with a minimum score of 85% within two attempts (*or as indicated by the instructor*).

Scoring: Divide the points earned by the total possible points. Failure to perform a critical step, indicated by an asterisk (*), results in grade no higher than an 84% (*or as indicated by the instructor*).

Time: Began_____ Ended_____ Total minutes: _____

Steps:	Point Value	Attempt 1	Attempt 2
Scenario #1: Role-play with a peer who will be the insurance representative. 1. Contact the patient's insurance company and verify the patient's eligibility for services. Provide the representative with the patient's information. Find out if the patient has a copayment for today's visit. Document the information obtained.	**20***		
Scenario #1 update: You need to provide the patient with the information that he owes a copayment for today's visit. 2. Inform the patient of his financial obligation of the copayment.	**10***		
Scenario update: He states he does not have the cash with him. 3. Inform the patient of the clinic policy regarding copayments and how the payment can be made.	**10**		
4. Demonstrate sensitivity and professionalism when discussing the payment. *(Refer to the Checklist for Affective Behaviors - Respect and Sensitivity)*	**15***		
Scenario #2: Role-play with a peer who will be the patient. 5. Determine the amount the patient owes by reviewing the patient's account record. Inform the patient the amount owed for services rendered.	**15***		
Scenario update: Patient states she does not have the money to pay the entire bill today. 6. Inform the patient of the clinic policy regarding overdue accounts and scheduling appointments. Provide the patient with options for the overdue amount based on the clinic policy.	**15**		
7. Demonstrate sensitivity and professionalism when discussing the payment and the situation. *(Refer to the Checklist for Affective Behaviors - Respect and Sensitivity)*	**15***		
Total Points	**100**		

Affective Behavior	Directions: Check behaviors observed during the role-play.					
Respect	**Negative, Unprofessional Behaviors**	**Attempt 1**	**Attempt 2**	**Positive, Professional Behaviors**	**Attempt 1**	**Attempt 2**
	Rude, unkind			Courteous, professional; assertive as required		
	Disrespectful, impolite			Polite, patient		
	Negative verbal communication (e.g., harsh words, disrespectful comments)			Professional verbal communication (e.g., respectful and understanding communication)		
	Brief, abrupt			Took time with person		
	Unconcerned with person's dignity			Maintained person's dignity		
	Negative nonverbal behaviors			Positive nonverbal behaviors		
	Other:			Other:		
Sensitivity	Distracted; not focused on the other person			Focused full attention on the other person		
	Judgmental attitude; not accepting attitude			Nonjudgmental, accepting attitude		
	Failed to clarify what the person verbally or nonverbally communicated			Used summarizing or paraphrasing to clarify what the person verbally or nonverbally communicated		
	Failed to acknowledge what the person communicated			Acknowledged what the person communicated		
	Rude, discourteous			Pleasant and courteous		
	Disregarded the person's dignity and rights			Maintained the person's dignity and rights		
	Other:			Other:		

Grading for Affective Behaviors		Point Value	Attempt 1	Attempt 2
Does not meet Expectation	• Response was insensitive and/or disrespectful. • Student demonstrated more than 2 negative, unprofessional behaviors during the interaction.	0		
Needs Improvement	• Response was insensitive and/or disrespectful. • Student demonstrated 1 or 2 negative, unprofessional behaviors during the interaction.	0		
Meets Expectation	• Response was sensitive and respectful; no negative, unprofessional behaviors observed. • More practice is needed for behavior to appear natural and for student to appear comfortable and at ease.	15		
Occasionally Exceeds Expectation	• Response was sensitive and respectful; no negative, unprofessional behaviors observed. • At times student appeared comfortable and at ease; but more practice is needed for behavior to become natural and consistent with a professional medical assistant.	15		
Always Exceeds Expectation	• Response was sensitive and respectful; no negative, unprofessional behaviors observed. • Student's behaviors appeared natural and comfortable. Behaviors are consistent with a professional medical assistant.	15		

Comments

CAAHEP Competencies	Step(s)
VII.P.3. Obtain accurate patient billing information	#1
VII.P.4. Inform a patient of financial obligations for services rendered	#2, 5
VII.A.1. Demonstrate professionalism when discussing patient's billing record	#4, 7
VII.A.2. Display sensitivity when requesting payment for services rendered	#4, 7
ABHES Competencies	**Step(s)**
7. Administrative Procedures c. Perform billing and collection procedures	Entire procedure

Procedure 19.3   Post Payments and Adjustments to Patient Account

Name _____   Date _____   Score _____

Task: To demonstrate sensitivity through verbal and nonverbal communication when discussing third-party requirements with patients.

Equipment and Supplies:
- Patient account ledger card or SimChart for the Medical Office software

Scenario: Monique Jones (06/23/1985) was seen 6 months ago for a wellness visit and lab work. Her insurance had lapsed, and she is completely responsible for the bill. She did not make any payments and resisted all attempts at collection of the balance of $172.00. Her account was turned over to the collection agency and they were able to collect the balance in full. The collection agency retains 50% of what they collect as payment. Post the collection agency payment and adjustment to her account.

Standard: Complete the procedure and all critical steps in _____ minutes with a minimum score of 85% within two attempts (*or as indicated by the instructor*).

Scoring: Divide the points earned by the total possible points. Failure to perform a critical step, indicated by an asterisk (*), results in grade no higher than an 84% (*or as indicated by the instructor*).

Time: Began_____   Ended_____   Total minutes: _____

Steps:	Point Value	Attempt 1	Attempt 2
1. Look up the ledger card for the patient account (or the patient ledger in SimChart). Confirm that you have the correct patient account.	30		
2. Post an adjustment to reverse the adjustment done when the account was turned over to the collection agency.	30		
3. Post the payment and adjustment that reflects the actual dollar amount received from the collection agency and the amount that was retained as payment.	40*		
Total Points	100		

Comments

CAAHEP Competencies	Step(s)
VII.P.1.b. Perform accounts receivable procedures to patient accounts including posting: payments	3
VII.P.1.c. Perform accounts receivable procedures to patient accounts including posting: adjustments	2, 3
ABHES Competencies	**Step(s)**
7. Administrative Procedures c. Perform billing and collection procedures	Entire procedure

Procedure 19.4   Prepare a Bank Deposit

Name _____   Date _____   Score _____

Task: Prepare a bank deposit for currency and checks.

Equipment and Supplies:
- Checks and currency for deposit (see scenario)
- Check for endorsement
- Calculator
- Paper method: bank deposit slip (Work Product 19.2)
- Electronic method: SimChart for the Medical Office (SCMO)

Scenario: The following checks need to be deposited:
- #3456 for $89
- #6954 for $136
- #9854-10 for $1366.65
- #8546 for $653.36
- #9865 for $890.22.

The following currency needs to be deposited:
- (19) $20 bills
- (10) $10 bills
- (46) $5 bills
- (73) $1 bills

The healthcare facility's name is Walden-Martin Family Medical Clinic, account number 123-456-78910, and the bank is Clear Water Bank, Anytown, Anystate.

Standard: Complete the procedure and all critical steps in _____ minutes with a minimum score of 85% within two attempts (*or as indicated by the instructor*).

Scoring: Divide the points earned by the total possible points. Failure to perform a critical step, indicated by an asterisk (*), results in grade no higher than an 84% (*or as indicated by the instructor*).

Time: Began_____ Ended_____ Total minutes: _____

Steps:	Point Value	Attempt 1	Attempt 2
1. Gather the documents to be used. For the electronic method, enter into the Simulation Playground in SCMO. Click on the Form Repository icon. On the INFO PANEL, click on Office Forms and then select Bank Deposit Slip.	10		
2. Add the date on the deposit slip.	10		
3. Using the calculator, calculate the amount of currency to be deposited. Enter the amount in the CURRENCY line, completing the dollar and cent boxes.	15*		
4. Enter the total amount in the TOTAL CASH line.	10		
5. For each check to be deposited, enter the check number, the dollars, and cents. List each check on a separate line.	10		

6.	Calculate the total to be deposited and enter the number in the TOTAL FROM ATTACHED LIST box.	15*		
7.	Enter the number of items deposited in the TOTAL ITEMS box.	10		
8.	Before completing the deposit slip, verify the check amounts listed and recalculate the totals. For the electronic method, click on SAVE.	10		
9.	Place a restrictive endorsement on the check(s).	10		
	Total Points	100		

Comments

CAAHEP Competencies	Step(s)
VII.P.2. Prepare a bank deposit	Entire procedure
ABHES Competencies	**Step(s)**
7. Administrative Procedures c. Perform billing and collection procedures	Entire procedure

Work Product 19.2 Bank Deposit Slip

DEPOSIT TICKET

WALDEN-MARTIN FAMLY MEDICAL CLINIC
1234 ANYSTREET
ANYTOWN, ANYSTATE 12345

DEPOSITS MAY NOT BE AVAILABLE FOR
IMMEDIATE WITHDRAWAL

Clear Water Bank
Anytown, Anystate

ACCOUNT NUMBER: 123-456-78910

Endorse & List Checks Separately

	Dollars	Cents
DATE _____		
CURRENCY		
COIN		
TOTAL CASH		
1.		
2.		
3.		
4.		
5.		
6.		
7.		
8.		
9.		
10.		
11.		
12.		
Less Cash Returned		
Total Items		Total Deposit		

Advanced Roles in Administration

CAAHEP	Assessments
V.C.3 Recognize barriers to communication	Skills and Concepts – D. 4
X.C.7.i. Define: risk management	Skills and Concepts – B. 2
X.C.10a Identify: Health Information Technology for Economic and Clinical Health (HITECH) Act	Skills and Concepts – F. 1

VOCABULARY REVIEW

Using the word pool on the right, find the correct word to match the definition. Write the word on the line after the definition.

1. The environment where something is created or takes shape; a base on which to build _____

2. Obeying, obliging, or yielding _____

3. Sticking together tightly _____

4. Evidence of authority, status, rights, entitlement to privileges _____

5. Contains all documents related to an individual's employment _____

6. To appoint a person as a representative _____

7. A term referring to actions taken by management to keep good employees _____

8. General _____

9. A steady employee whom a new staff member can approach with questions and concerns _____

10. Things that incite or spur to action; rewards or reasons for performing a task _____

11. Slighting; having a negative or degrading tone _____

12. Able to pay all debts _____

Word Pool
- consensus
- credential
- solvent
- matrix
- delegate
- incentive
- cohesive
- disparaging
- mentor
- retention
- human resources file
- compliant

SKILLS AND CONCEPTS

Answer the following questions. Write your answer on the line or in the space provided.

A. Medical Office Management

1. Describe the traits of a successful medical office manager. _____

    _____

    _____

    _____

    _____

    _____

    _____

2. Describe a good relationship between a manager and his or her employees._____

    _____

    _____

    _____

    _____

    _____

    _____

B. Office Management Responsibilities

1. List five office management responsibilities.

    a. _____

    b. _____

    c. _____

    d. _____

    e. _____

2. Define *risk management*. _____

    _____

    _____

    _____

    _____

C. Office Manager Role

1. List and define in your own words the five Cs of communication. _____

_____

_____

_____

_____

_____

2. List four characteristics of a good listener. _____

_____

_____

_____

_____

_____

3. Describe the ABC method of time management. _____

_____

_____

_____

_____

_____

D. Creating a Team Environment

1. What action improves communication in the healthcare workplace? _____

_____

_____

_____

2. Name two positive things that occur when communication improves in the healthcare workplace.

   a. _____

   b. _____

3. Name two actions an office manager can take to improve employee morale. _____

_____

_____

CERTIFICATION PREPARATION

Circle the correct answer.

1. Which is a quality of an effective leader or office manager?
   a. Has a sense of fairness
   b. Has good communication skills
   c. Uses good judgment
   d. All of the above

2. Something that spurs an individual to action or rewards an individual for performing a task is called
   a. morale.
   b. incentive.
   c. appraisal.
   d. circumvention.

3. Which act protects the employee against unsafe workplaces?
   a. Fair Labor Standards Act
   b. Family and Medical Leave Act
   c. Occupational Safety and Health Act
   d. Age Discrimination Act

4. Some managers assign a person to assist new employees during the initial probationary period; this person is called a
   a. mentor.
   b. supervisor.
   c. coworker.
   d. subordinate.

5. A group of employees who stick together during difficult times could be called
   a. cohesive.
   b. adaptive.
   c. affable.
   d. meticulous.

6. Which subjects cannot be discussed in a job interview?
   a. Religion
   b. Work history
   c. Previous terminations of employment
   d. None of the above

7. The process of inciting a person to some action or behavior is called
   a. reprimand.
   b. motivation.
   c. circumvention.
   d. appraisal.

8. Which is a strong method of improving employee morale and encouraging outstanding performance?
   a. Incentives
   b. Recognition
   c. Fraternizing with subordinates outside work
   d. All of the above

9. Which is critical for good communication and smooth operation of a medical facility?
   a. Scheduling activities that involve the families of employees
   b. Holding regular staff meetings and sending regular emails and memos
   c. Shielding employees from negative information
   d. All of the above

10. Which employee behavior is grounds for immediate dismissal without warning?
    a. Embezzlement
    b. Insubordination
    c. Violation of patient confidentiality
    d. All of the above

WORKPLACE APPLICATIONS

1. Create a job description or job posting for a "dream" job of your choice. Make sure to include the duties, required education, and other details typically found in postings.

_____

_____

_____

_____

_____

_____

_____

2. Create a plan of how to screen applications and résumés for a medical assistant job in a family practice department. Describe the process you would use to evidentially identify the few applicants who should be interviewed.

_____

_____

_____

_____

_____

_____

_____

_____

_____

_____

INTERNET ACTIVITIES

1. Using online resources, research team-building exercises designed to promote and build teamwork for a group of employees. Create a poster presentation, a PowerPoint presentation, or write a paper summarizing your research. Include the following points in your project:
   a. Describe three team-building activities.
   b. Why do you think each of these activities will promote and build teamwork?
   c. How would you make sure that these activities are relevant to working in healthcare?

2. Using online resources, research the I-9 form. Create a poster presentation, a PowerPoint presentation, or write a paper summarizing your research. Include the following points in your project:
   a. Describe the purpose of the form.
   b. Summarize the process for completing the I-9 form.
   c. Describe acceptable documentation used to complete the form.

Medical Emergencies

CAAHEP Competencies	Assessment
I.C.13. List principles and steps of professional/provider CPR	Skills and Concepts – B. 19
I.C.14. Describe basic principles of first aid as they pertain to the ambulatory healthcare setting	Skills and Concepts – B. 6, 8, 13, 14, 16
I.P.13.a. Perform first aid procedures for: bleeding	Procedure 21.5
I.P.13.b. Perform first aid procedures for: diabetic coma or insulin shock	Procedure 21.1
I.P.13.c. Perform first aid procedures for: fractures	Procedure 21.5
I.P.13.d. Perform first aid procedures for: seizures	Procedure 21.3
I.P.13.e. Perform first aid procedures for: shock	Procedure 21.6
I.P.13.f. Perform first aid procedures for: syncope	Procedure 21.5
I.A.1. Incorporate critical thinking skills when performing patient assessment	Procedure 21.2
X.P.3. Document patient care accurately in the medical record	Procedure 21.1 through 21.6

ABHES Competencies	Assessment
8. Clinical Procedures g. Recognize and respond to medical office emergencies	Procedure 21.1 through 21.7

VOCABULARY REVIEW

Using the word pool on the right, find the correct word to match the definition. Write the word on the line after the definition.

Group A

1. A catheter that is inserted into the trachea through the mouth; provides a patent airway _____
2. Open _____
3. A term used in healthcare settings to indicate an emergency situation and summon the trained team to the scene

   _____
4. A rolling supply cart that contains emergency equipment

   _____
5. A patient without an appointment _____
6. The level and type of care an ordinary, prudent healthcare professional having the same training and experience in a similar practice would have provided under a similar situation

   _____
7. Contraction of the muscles causing the narrowing of the inside tube of the vessel _____
8. The application of manual chest compressions and ventilations (also called *rescue breathing*) to patients who are not breathing or do not have a pulse; also known as *basic life support* (BLS)

   _____
9. A written flow map to make triage decisions; based on answers to questions, the person moves through the map until a triage decision is made _____
10. To sort out and classify the injured; used in the military and emergency settings to determine the priority of a patient to be treated _____

Word Pool
- triage flow map
- triage
- walk-in patient
- crash cart
- vasoconstriction
- cardiopulmonary resuscitation (CPR)
- standard of care
- endotracheal (ET) tube
- code
- patent

Group B

1. Tissue death _____
2. Redness _____
3. Itching _____
4. A position on the person's side that helps to keep the airway open and clear _____
5. A sensation that causes someone to feel as though everything is spinning _____
6. A traumatic brain injury caused by a blow to the head

   _____
7. A sudden increase of electrical activity in one or more parts of the brain _____
8. Also called a *stroke* _____
9. Also called *over breathing*; a rapid and deep breathing

   _____
10. Fainting _____

Word Pool
- seizure
- pruritus
- recovery position
- concussion
- syncope
- cerebrovascular accident
- necrosis
- vertigo
- erythema
- hyperventilation

ABBREVIATIONS
Write out what each of the following abbreviations stands for.

1. CPR _____

2. ET _____

3. LPN _____

4. RN _____

5. IV _____

6. AED _____

7. PPE _____

8. %TBSA _____

9. IM _____

10. RICE _____

11. CVA _____

12. ED _____

13. MI _____

14. EAP _____

15. POTS _____

SKILLS AND CONCEPTS
Answer the following questions. Write your answer on the line or in the space provided.

A. Emergency Equipment and Supplies

1. The following questions relate to crash carts.

    a. How often should a crash cart be checked? _____

    b. Who should check the crash cart? _____

    c. Describe how to check crash cart supplies. _____

    _____

    _____

2. List the equipment required when a provider performs an endotracheal tube intubation. _____

    _____

    _____

3. The following statements relate to common medications found on crash carts.

   a. _____ is used for bradycardia and will increase the heart rate.

   b. _____ is used for seizures.

   c. _____ is used for anaphylaxis, severe asthma, and cardiac arrest.

   d. _____ is an antihistamine that is used for allergic reactions.

   e. _____, a hormone that simulates the liver to release glucose into the blood, is given for hypoglycemia.

   f. _____ is used for opioid overdoses.

4. Describe the Broselow tape and Broselow ColorCode Cart. _____

   _____

   _____

B. Handling Emergencies

1. What is the role of the medical assistant with emergency situations? _____

   _____

2. Describe first aid procedures for the following conditions.

   a. Frostbite_____

   _____

   b. Hypothermia _____

   _____

   c. Heat cramps _____

   _____

   d. Heat exhaustion _____

   _____

   e. Heat stroke _____

   _____

   f. Minor burns _____

   _____

   g. Major burns _____

   _____

3. List six signs and symptoms of poisoning. _____

_____

4. Describe first aid procedures for poisoning. _____

_____

_____

5. Describe first aid procedures for severe allergic reactions. _____

_____

_____

6. What is the first aid procedure in the ambulatory care facility for an animal bite? _____

_____

7. What types of screening questions should a medical assistant ask a patient who is calling regarding an animal bite?

_____

_____

8. What is the first aid procedure for a foreign body in the eye and what is done in the ambulatory care facility?

_____

_____

9. _____ is called *severe hypoglycemia* or *insulin reaction*.

10. _____ is called *severe hyperglycemia*.

11. List five symptoms of hypoglycemia and two symptoms of severe hypoglycemia. _____

_____

_____

12. List five symptoms of hyperglycemia and two symptoms of diabetic ketoacidosis. _____

_____

_____

13. What are first aid procedures and additional treatments for insulin shock in a conscious and unconscious individual?

_____

_____

_____

_____

_____

_____

14. Describe how to splint an injured extremity. _____

_____

_____

15. Why is a cold pack applied to a musculoskeletal injury? _____

_____

16. For the following scenarios, the patient is in the ambulatory care facility. Describe first aid that the medical assistant should provide.

   a. A patient gets dizzy. _____

   _____

   _____

   b. A patient has seizure-like activity. _____

   _____

   _____

   c. A patient is confused and not making sense; has left arm and leg weakness and facial drooping.

   _____

   _____

   d. A patient is having an asthma attack._____

   _____

   _____

   e. A patient faints. _____

   _____

   _____

   f. A patient is bleeding from a gash on her arm. There is no obvious debris in the wound._____

   _____

   _____

17. A patient goes into shock. What is the typical treatment in the ambulatory care facility? _____

_____

_____

18. A patient has chest pain and left arm pain. What is the typical treatment in the ambulatory care facility?

_____

_____

19. Using Procedure 21.7, summarize the steps and principles involved with rescue breathing, CPR, and using the AED machine.

_____

_____

_____

_____

_____

_____

_____

CERTIFICATION PREPARATION

Circle the correct answer.

1. What is considered a mild heat-related illness that causes muscle pains and spasms due to electrolyte imbalance?
   a. Heat stroke
   b. Heat exhaustion
   c. Heat cramps
   d. Hypothermia

2. What is considered a partial-thickness burn?
   a. First-degree burn
   b. Second-degree burn
   c. Third-degree burn
   d. Fourth-degree burn

3. Which type of burn causes erythema, tenderness, and physical sensitivity, but no scar development occurs?
   a. First-degree burn
   b. Second-degree burn
   c. Third-degree burn
   d. Fourth-degree burn

4. An adult has burns on his back, left arm and hand, and left foot and leg. Using the Rule of Nines, estimate the percentage of total burn surface area.
   a. 18%
   b. 27%
   c. 36%
   d. 45%

5. Which animal is not a common carrier of rabies?
   a. Guinea pig
   b. Raccoon
   c. Bat
   d. Fox

6. What is a symptom of a concussion?
   a. Confusion and amnesia
   b. Ringing in the ears
   c. Temporary loss of consciousness right after the incident
   d. All of the above

7. What is a symptom of a cerebrovascular accident?
   a. Confusion and speech difficulty
   b. Numbness of the face, arm, or leg
   c. Problem seeing in one or both eyes
   d. All of the above

8. What is not a sign of a partial airway obstruction?
   a. Forceful or weak coughing
   b. Bluish skin color
   c. Labored, noisy, or gasping breathing
   d. Panicked appearance, extreme anxiety, or agitation

9. What is a possible cause of syncope?
   a. Dehydration
   b. Standing up too quickly
   c. Drop in blood glucose
   d. All of the above

10. What is not a typical symptom of a shock?
    a. Anxiety and agitation
    b. Chest pain
    c. Nausea
    d. Diaphoresis

Documentation

Comments

CAAHEP Competencies	Step(s)
I.P.13.b. Perform first aid procedures for: diabetic coma or insulin shock	Entire procedure
X.P.3. Document patient care accurately in the medical record	5
ABHES Competencies	**Step(s)**
8. g. Recognize and respond to medical office emergencies	Entire procedure

Procedure 21.2 Incorporate Critical Thinking Skills When Performing Patient Assessment

Name _____ Date _____ Score _____

Task: Use critical thinking skills while performing a patient assessment regarding a neurologic emergency.

Scenario: You are working with Dr. Martin, a family practice provider. Maude Crawford's daughter called concerned about her mother. She stated that Maude fell and hit her head. She was "knocked out" for about a minute. She has been acting differently since the fall. You need to follow the "Emergency Phone Protocol" for your clinic.

Directions: Role-play the scenario with a peer. The peer will be the daughter and you will be the medical assistant. The peer can make up information regarding the scenario. Your instructor will be the provider.

WMFM Clinic – Neurologic Emergency Phone Protocol:

Obtain the patient's name, date of birth, signs/symptoms, and the history of the situation. After call, document situation, symptoms, and action in the patient's health record.

With the following concerns, send the patient to the emergency department via the ambulance immediately.
- Seizure lasting 3 or more minutes
- Passing out or fainting; dizziness or weakness that doesn't go away
- Sudden or unusual headache that starts suddenly
- Unable to see or speak; sudden confusion
- Neck or spine injury
- Injuries that cause loss of feeling or inability to move
- Head injury with passing out, fainting, or confusion

With the following concerns, schedule a visit for the same day. If no appointments are available, consult the triage nurse or the provider regarding the situation.
- Headache/migraine
- Nonemergent neurologic concern

Equipment and Supplies:
- Patient's health record
- Paper and pen
- Emergency Phone Protocol for clinic

Standard: Complete the procedure and all critical steps in _____ minutes with a minimum score of 85% within two attempts (*or as indicated by the instructor*).

Scoring: Divide the points earned by the total possible points. Failure to perform a critical step, indicated by an asterisk (*), results in grade no higher than an 84% (*or as indicated by the instructor*).

Time: Began_____ Ended_____ Total minutes: _____

Steps:	Point Value	Attempt 1	Attempt 2
1. Write five questions that can be asked to obtain additional information on the patient's signs and symptoms.	20*		
Scenario update: Role-play the scenario with a peer. 2. Obtain the patient's name and date of birth.	10		
3. Write down the patient's information obtained.	20		
4. Using critical thinking skills, ask appropriate questions to obtain information about the patient's condition. *(Refer to the Checklist for Affective Behaviors.)*	15*		
5. Follow the protocol to determine what actions to take. *(Refer to the Checklist for Affective Behaviors.)*	15*		
6. Instruct the caller on what should be done.	10		
7. Document the call in the patient's health record. Include the caller's name, the patient's condition (e.g., signs, symptoms, and concerns), name of the protocol used, information given to the caller, and the provider who was notified.	10		
Total Points	100		

Checklist for Affective Behaviors

Affective Behavior	Directions: *Check behaviors observed during the role-play.*					
Critical Thinking	**Negative, Unprofessional Behaviors**	**Attempt** 1	**Attempt** 2	**Positive, Professional Behaviors**	**Attempt** 1	**Attempt** 2
	Coached or told of an issue or problem			Independently identified the problem or issue		
	Failed to ask relevant questions related to the condition			Asked appropriate questions to obtain the information required		
	Failed to consider alternatives; failed to ask questions that demonstrate understanding of principles/concepts			Willing to consider other alternatives; asked appropriate questions that showed understanding of principles/concepts		
	Failed to make an educated, logical judgment/decision; actions or lack of actions demonstrated unsafe practices and/or do not follow the protocol			Made an educated, logical judgment/decision based on the protocol; actions reflected principles of safe practice		
	Other:			Other:		

Grading for Affective Behaviors		Point Value	Attempt 1	Attempt 2
Does not meet Expectation	• Response fails to show critical thinking. • Student demonstrated more than 2 negative, unprofessional behaviors during the interaction.	0		
Needs Improvement	• Response fails to show critical thinking. • Student demonstrated 1 or 2 negative, unprofessional behaviors during the interaction.	0		
Meets Expectation	• Response demonstrates critical thinking; no negative, unprofessional behaviors observed. • More practice is needed for behavior to appear natural and for student to appear comfortable and at ease.	15		
Occasionally Exceeds Expectation	• Response demonstrates critical thinking; no negative, unprofessional behaviors observed. • At times student appeared comfortable and at ease; but more practice is needed for behavior to become natural and consistent with a professional medical assistant.	15		
Always Exceeds Expectation	• Response demonstrates critical thinking; no negative, unprofessional behaviors observed. • Student's behaviors appeared natural and comfortable. Behaviors are consistent with a professional medical assistant.	15		

Questions to ask

Documentation

Comments

CAAHEP Competencies	Step(s)
I.A.1. Incorporate critical thinking skills when performing patient assessment	Entire role-play
X.P.3. Document patient care accurately in the medical record	9
ABHES Competencies	**Step(s)**
8.g. Recognize and respond to medical office emergencies	Entire procedure

Procedure 21.3   Provide First Aid for a Patient with Seizure Activity

Name _____   Date _____   Score _____

Tasks: Provide first aid to an individual having seizure activity and document in the health record.

Scenario: You are working with Dr. Martin, a family practice provider. Walter Biller arrives for his appointment.

Directions: Read the scenario and role-play the situation with a peer. The peer will be the patient and you are the medical assistant.

Equipment and Supplies:
- Watch
- Folded towel, blanket, or coat
- Patient's health record
- Gloves and other personal protective equipment (as required)

Standard: Complete the procedure and all critical steps in _____ minutes with a minimum score of 85% within two attempts (*or as indicated by the instructor*).

Scoring: Divide the points earned by the total possible points. Failure to perform a critical step, indicated by an asterisk (*), results in grade no higher than an 84% (*or as indicated by the instructor*).

Time: Began_____ Ended_____ Total minutes: _____

Steps:	Point Value	Attempt 1	Attempt 2
1. Wash hands or use hand sanitizer.	5		
2. Greet the patient. Identify yourself. Verify the patient's identity with full name and date of birth.	10		
Scenario update: While you are getting Mr. Biller's health history, he starts to have seizure activity. 3. Lower the patient to the floor and note the time when the seizure started. Gently raise the chin to tilt the head back slightly to open the airway.	15		
4. Yell for help while moving the patient into the recovery position.	15		
5. Check his pulse rate and respiration rate.	15		
6. Apply gloves and other personal protective equipment as needed.	10		
7. Clear any hard or sharp items away from the patient. Place a soft folded towel, blanket, or coat under the patient's head.	10		
8. Remove the patient's glasses (if on) and loosen any constrictive clothing around the neck. Stay with the person until he or she is fully awake and continue to monitor the respiration and pulse rates.	10		
9. Document the first aid measures you provided in the order that they occurred. In addition, document the seizure activity seen, length of the episode, and the provider notified.	10		
Total Points	100		

Documentation

Comments

CAAHEP Competencies	Step(s)
I.P.13.d. Perform first aid procedures for: seizures	Entire procedure
X.P.3. Document patient care accurately in the medical record	9
ABHES Competencies	**Step(s)**
8.g. Recognize and respond to medical office emergencies	Entire procedure

Procedure 21.4   Provide First Aid for a Choking Patient

Name _____ Date _____ Score _____

Tasks: Provide first aid to a conscious adult who is choking. Document in the health record.

Scenario: You are working with Dr. Martin, a family practice provider. As you return from lunch, you notice that an adult visitor is having an issue. It appears that she had been eating fast food and now she is holding her neck with both hands. She appears to be panicking.

Directions: Read the scenario and role-play the situation with a peer. The peer will be the visitor and you are the medical assistant.

Equipment and Supplies:
- Patient's health record
- Gloves
- Mannequin

Standard: Complete the procedure and all critical steps in _____ minutes with a minimum score of 85% within two attempts (*or as indicated by the instructor*).

Scoring: Divide the points earned by the total possible points. Failure to perform a critical step, indicated by an asterisk (*), results in grade no higher than an 84% (*or as indicated by the instructor*).

Time: Began_____ Ended_____ Total minutes: _____

Steps:	Point Value	Attempt 1	Attempt 2
1. Approach the person and ask, "Are you choking?"	10		
Scenario update: She nods her head yes and cannot speak. She is standing. 2. Yell for help. Wear gloves if available. Stand behind the victim with your feet slightly apart. Reach your arms around the person's waist.	15*		
3. Make a fist and place it just above the person's navel. Make sure your thumb side is next to the person. Grasp the fist tightly with your other hand. *Note: Do not do abdominal thrusts on your peer.*	15*		
Scenario update: The next steps must be done on a mannequin. 4. With the correct hand position, make quick, upward and inward thrusts with your fist. Do five abdominal thrusts before doing back blows.	15*		
5. Stand behind the person and wrap one arm around the person's upper body. Position the person so he or she is bent forward with the chest parallel to the ground.	15		
6. Use the heel of your other hand to give a firm blow between the shoulder blades. Check to see if the object dislodges. If not, continue by giving another four back blows.	10		
7. Continue to give five abdominal thrusts followed by five back blows until the object is dislodged or the person loses consciousness. *Note:* If the person faints or loses consciousness, lower the person to the floor. Call 911 (or the local emergency number) or have someone else call. Begin CPR starting with chest compressions. Check to see if the item is in the airway. Only remove it if it is loose.	10		

Scenario update: After two sets, she coughs out a piece of food. She can now talk. 8. Arrange for the person to be seen by the provider. Document the first aid measures you provided in the order that they occurred.	**10**		
Total Points	**100**		

Documentation

Comments

ABHES Competencies	Step(s)
8.g. Recognize and respond to medical office emergencies	Entire procedure

Procedure 21.5 Provide First Aid for a Patient With a Bleeding Wound, Fracture, and Syncope

Name _____ Date _____ Score _____

Tasks: Provide first aid to an individual with a suspected fracture, a bleeding wound, and syncope. Document the first aid you provide.

Scenario: You are returning from lunch and see a person fall at the entrance of the healthcare facility. He is an older man and is complaining of pain in his right lower arm. His arm looks deformed and is bleeding. You call for help. A provider comes, and coworkers bring supplies. The provider tells you to care for the wound and splint the arm before moving the individual. You have a coworker helping you.

Directions: Read the scenario and role-play the situation with two peers. One peer will be the patient and the other peer will be a coworker. You will be the medical assistant.

Equipment and Supplies:
- Gloves
- Sterile gauze
- Bandage
- Splinting material (e.g., SAM splint)
- Coban wrap or gauze roll

Standard: Complete the procedure and all critical steps in _____ minutes with a minimum score of 85% within two attempts (*or as indicated by the instructor*).

Scoring: Divide the points earned by the total possible points. Failure to perform a critical step, indicated by an asterisk (*), results in grade no higher than an 84% (*or as indicated by the instructor*).

Time: Began_____ Ended_____ Total minutes: _____

Steps:	Point Value	Attempt 1	Attempt 2
1. Wash hands or use hand sanitizer if possible. Identify yourself to the patient. Obtain the patient's name and date of birth as you put on gloves.	10		
2. Using sterile gauze, apply direct pressure over the wound to stop the bleeding. Make sure to immobilize the injured arm as you apply pressure. If possible, elevate the arm to help slow the bleeding. If the blood seeps through the gauze, apply another layer of gauze on the initial one. Continue with the direct pressure until the bleeding stops.	15*		
3. Once the bleeding has stopped, cover the dressing with a bandage. Remember to immobilize the injured arm as you work.	10		
Scenario update: As you apply the bandage to the injured arm, the patient states he does not feel good. He says he feels dizzy and thinks he is going to pass out. Your peer takes over by supporting his arm, and the man faints. He is still breathing and has a pulse. 4. Position the patient on his back. Continue to check his respirations and pulse rates.	15*		
5. Loosen any constrictive clothing around the neck and chest. Raise the legs above the heart level (about 12 inches).	15*		

Scenario update: After a few minutes, he starts to come around. He jokes that blood makes him faint. As he is lying on his back talking with you, you need to splint his injured arm. 6. Use the splint material and shape it to the injured arm. Do not straighten the arm. Apply the splint beyond the joint above and the joint below the injury.	**15***		
7. Use Coban or a gauze roll to secure the splint in place. Encourage the patient to hold the injured arm against his chest as he moves.	**10***		
8. Document the first aid measures you provided in the order that they occurred. Indicate the provider was at the scene.	**10**		
Total Points	**100**		

Documentation

Comments

CAAHEP Competencies	Step(s)
I.P.13.a. Perform first aid procedures for: bleeding	2, 3
I.P.13.c. Perform first aid procedures for: fractures	6, 7
I.P.13.f. Perform first aid procedures for: syncope	4, 5
X.P.3. Document patient care accurately in the medical record	8
ABHES Competencies	**Step(s)**
8.g. Recognize and respond to medical office emergencies	Entire procedure

Procedure 21.6   Provide First Aid for a Patient With Shock

Name _____ Date _____ Score _____

Tasks: Provide first aid to an individual who is in shock. Document the first aid you provide.

Scenarios: You are working with Dr. Julie Walden. The administrative medical assistant at the reception desk notifies you that Robert Caudill (date of birth [DOB] 10/31/1940) is here and looks very ill. You bring the patient and his wife immediately back to the procedure room, as it is the only available room. He asks to move to the exam table and you assist him as he transfers to the table. You obtain his vital signs, which are: P: 92, R: 26, BP 72/48, and T: 103.2° F

Directions: Role-play the scenario with two peers. One peer will be the patient and the other peer will be the wife. You will be the medical assistant.

Equipment and Supplies:
- Stethoscope
- Watch
- Pen
- Sphygmomanometer (blood pressure cuff)
- Pillows, blankets, or small stool to help elevate the feet
- Exam table

Standard: Complete the procedure and all critical steps in _____ minutes with a minimum score of 85% within two attempts (*or as indicated by the instructor*).

Scoring: Divide the points earned by the total possible points. Failure to perform a critical step, indicated by an asterisk (*), results in grade no higher than an 84% (*or as indicated by the instructor*).

Time: Began_____ Ended_____ Total minutes: _____

Steps:	Point Value	Attempt 1	Attempt 2
1. Call for help. Monitor the patient's breathing and pulse until the provider arrives.	10		
Scenario update: The provider examines the patient and suspects septic shock. You administer 2 L of oxygen per nasal cannula as the provider ordered. The triage RN inserts an IV and administers IV fluids. The provider directs another medical assistant to call 911. 2. Raise the patient's legs 12 inches.	15*		
3. Make sure the patient's head is flat on the bed.	10*		
4. Loosen the person's clothing. Make sure the clothing does not restrict the neck and chest area.	15*		
5. Obtain a pulse rate, respiration rate, and blood pressure. Continue to monitor the patient's airway, pulse rate, and respiration rate.	15		
6. While monitoring the patient, speak calmly with the patient. Use a gentle tone of voice. Demonstrate a calming body language (e.g., do not appear scared, rushed, or out of control).	15		
7. Talk calmly with the patient's wife and explain what is occurring. Answer any questions the wife may have.	10		

8.	Document the first aid measures you provided in the order that they occurred. Indicate which provider examined the patient. In addition, document the administration of oxygen and the vital signs obtained.	10		
	Total Points	100		

Documentation

Comments

CAAHEP Competencies		**Step(s)**
I.P.13.e. Perform first aid procedures for: shock		Entire procedure
X.P.3. Document patient care accurately in the medical record		8
ABHES Competencies		**Step(s)**
8.g. Recognize and respond to medical office emergencies		Entire procedure

Procedure 21.7 Provide Rescue Breathing, Cardiopulmonary Resuscitation (CPR), and Automated External Defibrillator (AED)

Name _____ Date _____ Score _____

Tasks: Perform rescue breathing and CPR. Use the AED machine.

Scenario: You are out jogging and find a person on the ground. No one is around.

Directions: Role-play the scenario with a peer. The peer will be the person on the ground.

Equipment and Supplies:
- AED machine with adult pads
- Barrier ventilation device
- Mannequin
- Gloves (if available)

Standard: Complete the procedure and all critical steps in _____ minutes with a minimum score of 85% within two attempts (*or as indicated by the instructor*).

Scoring: Divide the points earned by the total possible points. Failure to perform a critical step, indicated by an asterisk (*), results in grade no higher than an 84% (*or as indicated by the instructor*).

Time: Began_____ Ended_____ Total minutes: _____

Steps:	Point Value	Attempt 1	Attempt 2
1. Check the scene for safety. Is it safe to approach and provide help to the victim?	5		
2. Check the person's response. Tap the individual on the shoulder and shout, "Are you all right?" Pause for a few moments for a response.	5		
Scenario update: There is no response from the individual. A bystander comes up and you direct that person to find an AED machine. 3. Call 911 and answer the questions from the dispatcher.	10		
4. Put on gloves if available. Roll the person over if the person is face down. Roll the person as an entire unit, supporting the head, neck and back. Open the airway and assess the respirations and the pulse for 5-10 seconds. **Note:** Occasional gasping is not considered breathing. • Person is breathing and has a pulse: If no head, neck, or spinal injury is suspected, then place the patient in the recovery position. • Person is not breathing and has a pulse: Give ventilations and monitor pulse. • Person is not breathing and has no pulse: Give CPR starting with compressions.	10*		

Scenario update: The individual has a weak pulse and is not breathing. (Use a mannequin for the following steps.) 5. Use a barrier device if available. Pinch the person's nose and give each rescue breath over 1 second. Watch for the chest to rise. Give the appropriate amount of ventilations for the person's age. Continue to monitor the pulse as you give rescue breaths. *Note:* For a situation in which a person had been choking, look in the mouth before giving a rescue breath. If you see the object, sweep it out with your finger. You can also provide nose ventilation, if the mouth is injured. Stoma ventilation must be done if the person has a stoma (in the throat area).	10*			
Scenario update: When you check the pulse again, there is no pulse. 6. Place your hands at the correct location on the chest. Bring your shoulders directly over the victim's sternum as you compress downward. Keep your elbows locked.	10			
7. Give 30 compressions at the appropriate depth. Give 100-120 compressions per minute.	10*			
8. Give two ventilations and watch for the chest to rise. Continue with the cycle.	10*			
Scenario update: After two cycles, a bystander brings an AED, but does not know how to use it. The bystander also does not know CPR. You need to stop the CPR and use the AED. 9. Turn on the AED and follow the directions. Attach the AED pads to the individuals' bare dry chest. Attach the pads to the machine if required. *Note:* Make sure to remove any medication patches and medication residue from the chest before operating applying the pads.	10*			
10. Have everyone stand back from the patient by announcing "Stand clear." Push the analyze button and allow the machine to analyze the heartbeat.	10*			

11.   Follow the prompts on the AED machine.
   a.   If a shock is advised, announce, "Stand clear" and make sure no one is touching the individual. Press the shock button. After the shock do CPR for 2 minutes starting with compressions. Continue following the prompts until the emergency responders arrive.
   b.   If a shock is not advised, continue doing CPR for 2 minutes starting with compressions. Continue following the prompts until the emergency responders arrive.
	10*			

Total Points	100			

Comments

ABHES Competencies	Step(s)
8.g. Recognize and respond to medical office emergencies	Entire procedure

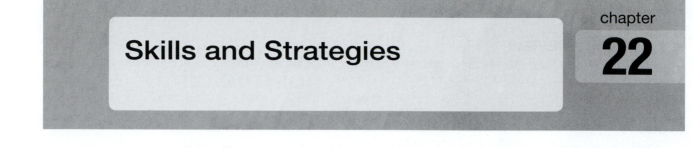

Skills and Strategies

chapter

22

CAAHEP Competencies	Assessment
X.C.9. List and discuss legal and illegal applicant interview questions	Skills and Concepts – J. 6; Certification Preparation – 7

ABHES Competencies	Assessment
10. Career Development a. Perform the essential requirements for employment, such as resume writing, effective interviewing, dressing professionally, time management, and following up appropriately	Procedure 22.1-22.6
b. Demonstrate professional behavior	Procedure 22.5, 22.6
c. Explain what continuing education is and how it is acquired	Certification Preparation – 10; Internet Activities – 3

VOCABULARY REVIEW

Using the word pool on the right, find the correct word to match the definition. Write the word on the line after the definition.

Group A

1. Allowing the listener to recap and review what was said

   _____

2. Rewording a statement to check the meaning and interpretation; also shows you are listening and understanding the speaker

   _____

3. The ability to communicate and interact with others; sometimes referred to as *soft skills* _____

4. Websites where employers post jobs; can be used by job seekers to identify open positions _____

5. Putting words to the patient's emotional reaction, which acknowledges the person's feelings _____

6. The act of working with another or other individuals

   _____

7. Allows the listener to get additional information

   _____

8. Exchange of information among others in your field

   _____

9. Being worthy of honor and respect from others

   _____

10. To have a deep awareness of another's suffering and the desire to lessen it _____

Word Pool
- job boards
- summarizing
- networking
- dignity
- paraphrasing
- interpersonal skills
- reflecting
- compassion
- collaboration
- clarification

Group B

1. A resume format that focuses on the person's employment history; useful when seeking employment in the same field as the education or experience _____

2. The most recent item is on top and the oldest item is last

   _____

3. A resume format that lists a person's abilities and skill sets and also includes the employment history _____

4. To read and mark corrections _____

5. Simulated; intended for imitation or practice

   _____

6. A resume format that is customized to a unique job posting

   _____

7. A person's abilities, skills, or expertise in an area

   _____

8. Return offer made by one who has rejected an offer or a job

   _____

Word Pool
- combination resume
- targeted resume
- counteroffer
- skill set
- reverse chronologic order
- proofread
- chronologic resume
- mock

ABBREVIATIONS
Write out what each of the following abbreviations stands for.

1. CPR _____

2. CMA _____

3. BLS _____

4. AAMA _____

5. RMA _____

6. AMT _____

7. CCMA_____

8. NHA _____

9. NCMA _____

10. NCCT _____

11. HIPAA _____

SKILLS AND CONCEPTS
Answer the following questions. Write your answer on the line or in the space provided.

A. Understanding Personality Traits Important to Employers

1. What traits help new employees blend with the existing staff? _____

    _____

    _____

2. List four interpersonal skills that are important for new employees to have._____

    _____

    _____

3. Describe effective verbal and nonverbal communication. _____

    _____

    _____

4. List four traits of effective nonverbal communication._____

    _____

    _____

5. Describe why listening to others is important._____

    _____

F. Developing a Resume

1. What is the purpose of a resume? _____

_____

_____

2. List three types of resumes and describe why each is used. _____

_____

_____

3. Describe information found in the education section of a resume. _____

_____

_____

4. Describe the work experience information required for all three types of resume. _____

_____

_____

5. How many years of employment history should be included in the resume? _____

6. What information should be included for certifications? _____

_____

_____

7. Describe how to create a visually appealing resume. _____

_____

_____

_____

_____

G. Developing a Cover Letter

1. What is the goal of a cover letter? _____

_____

_____

2. What two things can be done to help identify errors in a cover letter? _____

_____

_____

_____

3. What specific position information should appear in the cover letter? _____

_____

_____

H. Completing Online Profiles and Job Applications

1. What are the advantages of online profiles over paper applications for both the applicant and the employer?

_____

_____

_____

2. Describe four types of information required for online profiles and paper applications. _____

_____

_____

_____

_____

3. Describe the professional way to obtain references. _____

_____

_____

4. List three types of people that should be included on the reference list. _____

_____

_____

I. Creating a Career Portfolio

1. Describe the purpose of a career portfolio. _____

_____

_____

2. Describe materials you could include in a career portfolio. _____

_____

_____

_____

_____

_____

J. Job Interview

1. What are the four things a job seeker must do to prepare for an interview?_____

    _____

    _____

    _____

2. Why is it important to research the facility prior to the interview? _____

    _____

3. Describe what your interview attire would be like. _____

    _____

4. List six items to bring to an interview. _____

    _____

    _____

    _____

5. Explain how you would answer this question during an interview: "Tell me about yourself." _____

    _____

    _____

6. List six topics that might be discussed during an interview. For each topic, provide a legal and illegal question that addresses the topic. Use the book examples as a guide and come up with your own questions.

    _____

    _____

    _____

    _____

    _____

    _____

7. How should a person treat a phone interview? _____

    _____

    _____

8. Just prior to the interview starting, list three things an interviewee should do._____

    _____

    _____

9. Discuss the importance of good eye contact during an interview. _____

_____

_____

_____

10. Describe the importance of sending a thank-you note after an interview. _____

_____

_____

_____

K. You Got the Job!

1. Describe five ways a medical assistant can be successful in a new job. _____

_____

_____

_____

_____

2. Describe the 180-degree style performance appraisal. _____

_____

_____

_____

_____

3. Describe the 360-degree style performance appraisal. _____

_____

_____

_____

_____

4. When leaving a job, how soon should you give notice? _____

_____

CERTIFICATION PREPARATION

Circle the correct answer.

1. _____ means to have a deep awareness of another's suffering and a desire to lessen it.
   a. Interpersonal skills
   b. Reflecting
   c. Compassion
   d. Dignity

2. "Communicates well" is a _____.
   a. technical skill
   b. personality trait
   c. transferable job skill
   d. both a and b

3. What is the best and most effective way to find employment?
   a. Checking job boards and newspaper ads
   b. Using the school career placement office
   c. Networking and checking job boards
   d. Using employment agencies

4. Which is the most popular type of resume that is used when people are seeking employment in the same field as their education or experience?
   a. Reverse chronologic
   b. Chronologic
   c. Combination
   d. Targeted

5. What is true regarding the header in the resume and cover letter?
   a. The information should appear on all pages of the cover letter and resume
   b. Contains the person's name and mailing address
   c. Contains a phone number and a professional email address
   d. All of the above are true

6. Which item is typically presented in a reverse chronologic order on a resume?
   a. Education information
   b. Work experience
   c. Skills
   d. Both a and b

7. What is an illegal interview question?
   a. "Are you eligible to work in this state?"
   b. "Who looks after your children when you work?"
   c. "Are you able to work 8 AM to 3 PM on the weekends?"
   d. "Have you ever been convicted of a federal offense?"

8. Form _____ is the Employee's Withholding Allowance Certificate.
   a. W-3
   b. W-2
   c. I-9
   d. W-4

9. Form _____ is the Employment Eligibility Verification Form.
   a. W-3
   b. W-2
   c. I-9
   d. W-4

10. What is the importance of continuing education for a medical assistant?
    a. Helps with keeping updated and current
    b. Needed to maintain a certification or registration
    c. Important for professional development
    d. All of the above

WORKPLACE APPLICATIONS

1. Select six interview questions from Figure 22.8 and write a response for each question. Your answer
    should be at least five sentences in length.

    _____

    _____

    _____

    _____

    _____

    _____

    _____

    _____

2. During an interview, Michelle was asked her age. Michelle knew this was not a legal interview question.
    If you were in this situation, how would you respond?

    _____

    _____

    _____

INTERNET ACTIVITIES

1. Using appropriate online resources, research one of the four national certification exams:
    *   Certified Medical Assistant (CMA) through the American Association of Medical Assistants
        (AAMA)
    *   Registered Medical Assistant (RMA) through the American Medical Technologists (AMT)
    *   Medical Assistant Certification (CCMA) through the National Healthcareer Association
    *   Medical Assistant (NCMA) through the National Center for Competency Testing (NCCT)

    In a PowerPoint, poster, or paper, address the following points:
    a. List the credential and the sponsoring agency
    b. Describe the exam (e.g., number of questions, coverage of topics, time limit)
    c. Describe the registration process
    d. Describe the requirements for maintaining the credential (e.g., continuing education, fees, retaking
        the exam)

2. Using online resources, identify four potential job openings that interest you. Describe each position in a
    brief paper and provide the websites for the openings.

3. Using online resources, identify two resources for continuing education for medical assistants. Briefly
    describe the resources and list the websites.

4. Using online resources, identify 8-10 potential job postings that interest you.

Procedure 22.1 Prepare a Chronologic Resume

Name _____ **Date** _____ **Score** _____

Task: Write an effective resume for use as a tool in obtaining employment.

Equipment and Supplies:
- Computer with word processing software and a printer
- Current job posting
- Resume paper
- Paper and pen

Standard: Complete the procedure and all critical steps in _____ minutes with a minimum score of 85% within two attempts (*or as indicated by the instructor*).

Scoring: Divide the points earned by the total possible points. Failure to perform a critical step, indicated by an asterisk (*), results in grade no higher than an 84% (*or as indicated by the instructor*).

Time: Began _____ **Ended** _____ **Total minutes:** _____

Steps:	Point Value	Attempt 1	Attempt 2
1. Apply critical thinking skills as you create a list of the personality traits (wanted by employers), technical skills, and transfer job skills that you possess. Also write down your career goal(s).	5		
2. Using the current job posting, identify the required and recommended qualifications and credentials needed for the position.	10		
3. Using the computer with word processing software, create a professional-looking header for your document. Include your name, address, telephone number(s), and email address. Select an appropriate font style for your name and a smaller font size for your contact information.	10		
4. Create a section header for "Education." For the learning institution(s) you attended, list the school's name, city and state, degree obtained, or coursework successfully completed, and the year. Include any additional educational information, such as grade point average (GPA), awards, and practicum information.	10		
5. Create a section header for "Healthcare Experience" and/or "Work Experience." Provide details about your work experience, including the facility's name, city and state, title of your position, start and end date (month and year), and job duties. The job duties must start with an active verb using the appropriate tense (e.g., a past job would have past tense verbs and a current job would include present tense verbs).	10		
6. Create a section header for "Special Skills" and list your special language skills, computer proficiencies, and other unique skills you possess that relate to the position.	10		
7. Create a section header for "Certifications and Credentials" and list the active credentials and certifications you have. Include the title of the certification, awarding agency, and the expiration date.	10		
8. All information on the resume needs to appear in reverse chronologic order (newest information is on top). Work experience should include both the start and end month and year.	10		

9.	The resume needs to look professional and interesting. Utilize font styles (e.g., bold, underline, italic) to emphasize important words and phrases. Use professional-looking bullets to list job duties and other information. Use keywords from the posting throughout the resume.	**15***		
10.	Proofread the resume. Correct any spelling, grammar, punctuation, or sentence structure errors you find. If time allows, have another person review the resume and use the feedback to revise your resume.	**10**		
	Total Points	**100**		

Comments

ABHES Competencies	Step(s)
10.a. Perform the essential requirements for employment, such as resume writing, effective interviewing, dressing professionally, time management, and following up appropriately	Entire procedure

Procedure 22.2 Create a Cover Letter

Name _____ Date _____ Score _____

Task: Write an effective cover letter that will accompany the resume.

Equipment and Supplies:
- Computer with word processing software and a printer
- Current job posting
- Resume paper
- Pen

Standard: Complete the procedure and all critical steps in _____ minutes with a minimum score of 85% within two attempts (*or as indicated by the instructor*).

Scoring: Divide the points earned by the total possible points. Failure to perform a critical step, indicated by an asterisk (*), results in grade no higher than an 84% (*or as indicated by the instructor*).

Time: Began_____ Ended_____ Total minutes: _____

Steps:	Point Value	Attempt 1	Attempt 2
1. Using the job posting, read through the job description. With a pen, circle the position requirements and the key phrases.	5		
2. Using the computer with word processing software, create a professional-looking header in the document's header that matches your resume header. Include your name, address, telephone number(s), and email address.	10		
3. Type the date in the correct location using the correct format. Have one blank line between the date line and the last line of the letterhead.	10		
4. Type the inside address using the correct spelling, punctuation, and location for the information. Leave 1 to 9 blank lines between the date and the inside address, depending on the location of the body of the letter.	10		
5. Starting on the second line below the inside address, type the salutation using the correct format. Use a colon after the person's name.	10		
6. Type the message in the body of the letter using the proper location and format. There should be a blank line after the salutation and between each paragraph. The message should be clear, concise, and professional. Use proper grammar, punctuation, capitalization, and sentence structure.	10		
7. The first paragraph should contain the title and number of the job posting. The middle paragraph(s) should summarize your strengths and include key phrases from the posting. The final paragraph should discuss your availability for an interview. The body should end with an expression of gratitude to the reader.	10		
8. Type a proper closing, leaving one blank line between the last line of the body and the closing. Use the correct format and location.	10		
9. Type the signature block using the correct format and location. There should be four blank lines between the closing and the signature block.	10*		
10. Spell-check and proofread the document. Check for proper tone, grammar, punctuation, capitalization, and sentence structure. Check for proper spacing between the parts of the letter.	10		

Work Product 22.1   Job Application

To be used with Procedure 22.3.

Name _____   **Date** _____   **Score** _____

WALDEN-MARTIN
FAMILY MEDICAL CLINIC
1234 ANYSTREET | ANYTOWN, ANYSTATE 12345
PHONE 123 123 1234 | FAX 123 123 5678

APPLICATION FOR EMPLOYMENT

Walden-Martin Family Medical Clinic is an equal opportunity employer and upholds the principles of equal opportunity employment. It is the policy of Walden-Martin Family Medical Clinic to provide employment, compensation and other benefits related to employment based on qualifications and performance, without regard to race, color, religion, national origin, age, sex, veteran status or disability, or any other basis prohibited by federal or state law. As an equal opportunity employer, Walden-Martin Family Medical Clinic intends to comply fully with all federal and state laws, and the information requested on this application will not be used for any purpose prohibited by law. Disabled applicants may request any needed accommodation. Please complete this application using ink, answer all questions completely, and sign the application.

Date: _____

Name: (First, Middle Initial, Last) _____

Social Security No.:_____   Phone: _____

Address:_____

City, State, Zip: _____

Have you been previously employed by Walden-Martin Family Medical Clinic?
☐ Yes ☐ No
If "Yes", when and job title?

How did you learn of the position for which you are applying?
☐ Newspaper/Print Advertisement ☐ Friend/Relative ☐ Employment Agency
☐ Job Service
☐ Radio/TV Advertisement ☐ Clinic Staff Person Name:

EMPLOYMENT DESIRED

Position(s) applied for: _____

☐ Full-time ☐ Part-time (If "Part time", number of shifts/hours desired _____)

Date available to start: _____ Salary requested: _____

PERSONAL HISTORY

Are you a United States citizen or do you have an entry permit which allows you to lawfully work in the U.S.? ☐ Yes ☐ No
    If applicable, Visa Type: _____ Immigration No.: _____

Are you at least 18 years old? ☐ Yes ☐ No

Are you ineligible to be employed with an AnyState licensed health care entity as a result of being found guilty by a court of law for abusing, neglecting, or mistreating individuals in a health care related setting? ☐ Yes ☐ No
    If "Yes," please explain: _____

Are you able to perform all of the duties required by the position for which you are applying, without endangering yourself or compromising the safety, health, or welfare of the patients or other staff member? ☐ Yes ☐ No
    If "No," please explain:_____

EDUCATION

	Name, City, State	Graduation Date	Course of Study/ Degree Obtained
High School:			
College:			
Other:			

LICENSURE/CERTIFICATION/REGISTRATION

Type of Certification, License or Registration	Agency/State	Registration Name

List any special skills or qualifications which you possess and feel are relevant to health care and the position for which you are applying.

_____

_____

_____

_____

_____

MILITARY SERVICE

From: _____   To: _____

Branch: _____

Duties: _____

Did you receive any specialized training? ☐ Yes   ☐ No
If "Yes", describe: _____

EMPLOYMENT HISTORY

Please give accurate and complete information. Start with present or most recent employer.
May we contact and communicate with your present employer? ☐ Yes   ☐ No

Employer:		Phone:	
Address:		**Supervisor:**	
Employed	Start: Month/Year: _____ Ended: Month/Year: _____	**Hourly Pay:**	Start: _____ Ended: _____
Position title and responsibilities:			
Reason for leaving:			

Employer:		Phone:	
Address:		**Supervisor:**	
Employed	Start: Month/Year: _____ Ended: Month/Year: _____	**Hourly Pay:**	Start: _____ Ended: _____
Position title and responsibilities:			
Reason for leaving:			

Employer:		Phone:	
Address:		Supervisor:	
Employed	Start: Month/Year: _____ Ended: Month/Year: _____	Hourly Pay:	Start: _____ Ended: _____
Position title and responsibilities:			
Reason for leaving:			

Employer:		Phone:	
Address:		Supervisor:	
Employed	Start: Month/Year: _____ Ended: Month/Year: _____	Hourly Pay:	Start: _____ Ended: _____
Position title and responsibilities:			
Reason for leaving:			

REFERENCES

Names of co-workers (no relatives) you have worked with and whom we may contact for a reference.

Name:	
Address:	
Phone:	
Job Title:	

Name:	
Address:	
Phone:	
Job Title:	

Name:	
Address:	
Phone:	
Job Title:	

Please read the following statements completely and carefully before you sign your name.

The Applicant HEREBY CERTIFIES that the answers given on this Application For Employment, including any statements or answers provided by the Applicant during interview, are true and correct. The Applicant fully authorizes Walden-Martin Family Medical Clinic to contact any references, past and present employers, persons, schools, law enforcement agencies and any other sources of information which may be relevant to the Applicant and this Application For Employment. It is understood and agreed that any misrepresentation, false statement, or omission by the Applicant will be sufficient reason for rejection of the Application For Employment or for dismissal from employment at any time, without recourse or liability to Walden-Martin Family Medical Clinic.

I have read, understand and agree to the above statement.

Sign: _____

Date: _____

Procedure 22.5   Practice Interview Skills During a Mock Interview

Name _____ **Date** _____ **Score** _____

Tasks: Project a professional appearance during a job interview and to be able to express the reasons the medical assistant is the best candidate for the position.

Equipment and Supplies:
- Current job posting
- Resume
- Cover letter
- Interview portfolio (optional)
- Application (optional)
- Interviewer
- Mock interview questions

Standard: Complete the procedure and all critical steps in _____ minutes with a minimum score of 85% within two attempts (*or as indicated by the instructor*).

Scoring: Divide the points earned by the total possible points. Failure to perform a critical step, indicated by an asterisk (*), results in grade no higher than an 84% (*or as indicated by the instructor*).

Time: Began_____ Ended_____ Total minutes: _____

Steps:	Point Value	Attempt 1	Attempt 2
1. Wear interview-appropriate attire and be groomed professionally.	15		
2. Portray a professional image by shaking hands firmly prior to the start of the interview. Ensure that each interviewer has a copy of your resume and cover letter. Refrain from nervous behaviors (e.g., saying "um", tapping a pen or your foot) during the interview.	10		
3. Answer introductory questions by providing only professional information. This may include information about your education, experience, and career goals.	10		
4. Answer interview questions with open, honest, and positive responses. Completely answer questions, provide information or examples, and do not answer in single sentences or with limited responses.	25		
5. Use key words from the job posting when answering the interview questions.	10		
6. Ask the interviewer two to three appropriate questions about the facility or the position.	20		
7. Express interest in the job and politely complete the interview by shaking hands and thanking the interviewer for the opportunity for the interview.	10		
Total Points	100		

Comments

ABHES Competencies	Step(s)
10.a. Perform the essential requirements for employment, such as resume writing, effective interviewing, dressing professionally, time management, and following up appropriately	Entire procedure

Procedure 22.6 Create a Thank-You Note for an Interview

Name _____ Date _____ Score _____

Task: Create a meaningful thank-you note to be sent after the interview process.

Equipment and Supplies:
- Computer with word processing software and a printer
- Job description
- Contact name from interview

Standard: Complete the procedure and all critical steps in _____ minutes with a minimum score of 85% within two attempts (*or as indicated by the instructor*).

Scoring: Divide the points earned by the total possible points. Failure to perform a critical step, indicated by an asterisk (*), results in grade no higher than an 84% (*or as indicated by the instructor*).

Time: Began_____ Ended_____ Total minutes: _____

Steps:	Point Value	Attempt 1	Attempt 2
1. Using word processing software, compose a professional letter using the business letter format. Include all of the required elements in the letter. Use correct spacing between the elements.	30		
2. Emphasize the particulars of the interview in the body of the letter.	20		
3. Include positive information you wish you had covered in the interview.	20		
4. Create a message that is concise and to the point.	20		
5. Proofread the letter and make any revisions as needed. Sign and send the thank-you note.	10		
Total Points	100		

Comments

ABHES Competencies	Step(s)
10.a. Perform the essential requirements for employment, such as resume writing, effective interviewing, dressing professionally, time management, and following up appropriately	Entire procedure

Notes

Notes

Notes

Notes

Notes